Wang-puh Wei and Chris Evans

Translated by Don McGinnis

Erotic Chinese Massage

The Sexy Secrets of Taoist Teachers

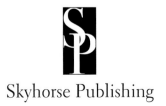

Skyhorse Publishing

This book offers suggestions only, and in no way should it be used as a substitute for consultation with professional therapists. The information provided in this work offers you the knowledge so you can choose, at your own risk, to act on that knowledge.

Original Title: Masaje Erótico Chino
© 1999, 2003, Editorial Océano, S.L.
(Barcelona, Spain)

English translation © 2015 by Skyhorse Publishing

Skyhorse Publishing books may be purchased in bulk at special discounts for sales promotion, corporate gifts, fund-raising, or educational purposes. Special editions can also be created to specifications. For details, contact the Special Sales Department, Skyhorse Publishing, 307 West 36th Street, 11th Floor, New York, NY 10018 or info@skyhorsepublishing.com.

Skyhorse® and Skyhorse Publishing® are registered trademarks of Skyhorse Publishing, Inc.®, a Delaware corporation.

Visit our website at www.skyhorsepublishing.com.

10 9 8 7 6 5 4 3 2 1

Library of Congress Cataloging-in-Publication Data is available on file.

Illustrations: Carles Baró

Cover design by Qualcom
Cover photo credit courtesy of Thinkstock

ISBN: 978-1-63220-324-3
Ebook ISBN: 978-1-63220-857-6

Printed in China

Contents

Harmony and eroticism

The movement of Tao is to go back;
The use of Tao is to accept.
All things come from the Tao.
The Tao comes from nothing.

Sexual energy is the energy of creation. It is the purest form of energy that humans possess and the only one that is capable of creating life. In any case, there are other possibilities. When procreation is not the goal, sexual energy is able to transform and open channels within the body to caches of energy that, for some reason, remain dormant inside us and prevent energy from flowing throughout the whole organism. Finding the balance between mind and body is one of the core ways of feeling good with ourselves and with our surroundings.

According to the *Tao*, the earth and the heavens sustain a permanent sexual union, which maintains balance. Because of this, it is essential that man and woman enter into communion with the cosmos and channel their energy to obtain health and pleasure.

The Taoist philosophy means freedom

According to Taoism, the mind and body must be in harmony. Sexuality and spirituality are inseparable. Taoism does not prohibit any form of sexual activity; on the contrary, it seeks to find lost harmony through the act of love. Sexual energy empowers emotions and shapes them until they become a rejuvenating and healing

The Taoist philosophy

The movement of the Tao is to return.
The effect of the Tao is flexibility.
All things in the universe are born from being.
Being is born from non being.

The *Tao*

Taoism is one of the oldest religions of China. It is based on the *Tao*, or absolute, that is the force or primordial reason for the universe and the cause of everything's existence. *Tao* teaches us to disregard all things, value life itself, and break the ties that bind us to the material world and the rest of mankind that disrupt the path to a pure life in communion with nature.

The concept of Taoism as a philosophy is attributed to Lao Tse, who is said to have been born in the year 571 B.C. His doctrine is based on the idea that *Tao is the life force of everything and the energy of both animate and inanimate objects*. Lao Tse established the path as a way to achieve an inner state of emptiness and repose and to avoid falling for the seductions of external things. He created a flexible and dynamic religion that adapts to social change throughout time.

The Book of Tao is a difficult philosophical work that, according to translations, takes one feeling or another. Due to its range, depth, and diversity of points of view, that feeling may not be unique. This book combines the teachings of Lao Tse and the Taoist practices of some of the greatest masters in a way so the world of *Tao* may open itself little by little to the reader. At times, and at first glance, some of the phrases in *The Book of Tao* may seem unconnected, but taking time to consider the meaning of each phrase is the proper way to understand *Tao* as a whole and not just individual concepts. All the same, in this work the approach is natural and will come about with practice.

Lao Tse's *The Book of Tao*

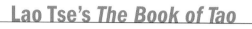

> In order to understand the richness and complexities of *The Book of the Tao*, one need only read this beautiful paragraph:
>
> The Tao that can be known is not the Tao.
> The substance of the world is only one name for the Tao.
> Tao is everything that exists and could exist.
> The world is but a map of what exists and could exist.
>
> External experiences serve as a way to feel the world,
> and internal experiences serve to understand it.
> Both kinds of experiences are the same within the Tao;
> they are different only among men.
> No experience may contain the Tao,
> which is infinitely larger and more subtle than the world.

Tao for men and women. In many previous works concerning *Tao* and sex, teachings have been targeted toward men. In those works, it is easy to forget that women are also able to enjoy sex from their perspective and that *Tao* contains important feminine traditions, as well.

These women were known in Chinese tradition as White Tigresses, and they were able to achieve a high degree of sexual and spiritual elevation. This allowed them to reach the height of their female potential and maintain their youth and beauty. (Editor's note: There is an excellent book regarding White Tigresses

10

written by Hsi Lai.) At present, there are only a few White Tigresses left in Taiwan, and they are struggling to keep this wisdom from fading. The White Tigresses employ spiritual and sexual methods to conserve their vigor and obtain immortality. Additionally, there were women that nurtured Taoism as nuns and practiced, as the men did, celibacy and rigorous meditation.

Chinese society was initially matriarchal, meaning that it was not strange to see many women practicing Taoism. When the moralists and Confucians imposed their own points of view, there were lineages of women, and also men, that kept the tradition alive. No other culture in history has so clearly seen that women are the incarnation of spiritual power and men of physical power.

Chinese culture understood perfectly that poorly channeled sex could be a source of illness, weakness, age, and death but that when used correctly, it could also become a great positive force that leads to health, vitality, longevity, and even immortality.

Feminine and masculine traditions

"When water and fire repeatedly intertwine within the Portal of the Heavens and melt into the cauldron, the divine elixir is made."

Water represents woman and fire is man,
the eternals of the *Yin* and *Yang*.

Stillness, the greatest principal of Taoism. "Sitting still while doing nothing" produces mental calmness and clarity. This spiritual state allows for the distinction between desires that are real and those that are not. It allows one to recognize man's basic needs rather than those imposed upon him by television and publicity. It makes it possible to empty the mind and make space for intuition.

The time has come, then, to remember "the path of nature," as put forth by Taoism. Its greatest principal is *ching-jing wu-wei* ("sitting while doing nothing"). In order to use it, we must forget all our Western prejudices, as doing nothing is considered a sin in Western civilization and where a person who is inactive is useless to society and thereby a nuisance. But we should not lose sight of the fact that even though the body remains still and apparently at rest, the mind may travel swiftly.

When one stops walking in order to reflect upon life itself, it is not hard to see how we are immersed in a multitude of artificial desires that lead us to fall into excess and deprive us of a light and harmonic life.

Among all the roads that man may follow during his life, Taoism takes the natural path, the principles of which are *sincerity with one's self* (working from within, without cause or external goals, without observing others, nor demanding attention), *self-discipline* (forcing oneself to do as desired), *spontaneity* and *balance*, and the *harmony of opposites* (the principle of the balanced middle).

Yin and Yang

According to the cosmological concepts elaborated on through Chinese philosophy, everything in nature, including man, is made up of *Yin* and *Yang*. All natural phenomena are caused by the interaction between both of these cosmic forces. *Tao* is considered in antiquity as the method of communication between *Yin* and *Yang* and thereby also represents harmony and the balance between man and woman, the sky and the earth, and all other dualities that exist in the world.

Yin is heavy, impure, and favors the earth. *Yang* is light, pure, and favors the sky. *Yin* is associated with darkness, passiveness, receptiveness, flexibility, softness, contraction, inwardness, downwardness, women, water, earth, and night. *Yang* is associated with light, activity, resistance, toughness, expansion, men, fire, sky, day, upwardness, and outwardness.

Yin and *Yang* are contrary but not exclusive, and they exist within everything around us. Both transform each other constantly, a natural tendency that becomes suppressed by homeostasis, a process that seeks to achieve balance through the use of regulatory mechanisms. If we place two receptacles on either side of a porous wall and in one of them we pour an acidic solution and in the other a basic solution, given time, the excess of acid becomes basic and vice versa, thereby balancing the whole system and creating a neutral solution.

Nature has a tendency to regulate its unbalances. So when there is an excess of *Yin*, it becomes *Yang* and vice versa. Just as Liu Tzu said:

> When *Yang* has reached its highest point, *Yin* begins to surge, and when *Yin* reaches its greatest height, it begins to to decline, and when the moon has grown to its greatest size, it starts to shrink. When the forces have reached their climax, they begin to weaken and when all things in nature have completely gathered together, they begin to spread out. Following the peak of each year is a downward spiral, and the most intense joys are followed by sadness. This is also the immutable condition of man.

This interaction between *Yin* and *Yang* can be understood perfectly through the following image: *Yin* contains in its interior the seed of *Yang* (the potential to become *Yang*), and *Yang* holds the seed of *Yin*. *Yin-Yang* is the polar and ever-changing dynamic that exists in all things.

The symbol of *Yin-Yang* is a representation of the cosmos. It contains the cycle of the Sun, the four seasons, twenty-four segments, and is the base of the *I Ching* and the Chinese calendar. The separation of both halves is sinusoidal, making it impossible to trace a diameter that divides the circle into two halves composed entirely of one color each. Inside each half, the other half is represented by a dot, indicating that all things contain both parts.

The constant transformations between *Yin* and *Yang* are what produce all natural phenomena. All its elements are related to one another, and in each relation there is a part of *Yin* and a part of *Yang*. The changes produced by this relationship are always an effort to bring both parts into balance.

Sexually speaking, man is *Yang* and woman is *Yin*, but both man and woman are part of both *Yin* and *Yang*. No being is only

Yin or only *Yang* by themselves but part of their surroundings. Said qualities belong not to the elements but to the relationship that is established among them and to the natural phenomena.

Yin and *Yang* are two opposite forces in constant shift. When the unity between them is broken, there emerges war, sickness, natural catastrophes, inequalities and injustices.

Just as when the relationship between two things tends toward balance, so does the relationship between *Yin* and *Yang* seek stability within that same object (the excess of one becomes regulated by the transformation of the other and vice versa). In man, this balance is called health. Traditional Chinese medicine classifies sickness according to the excess or lack of *Yin* or *Yang* within a determined meridian. Sexual pleasure can also help balance *Yin* and *Yang* within a person and thereby help their health to improve. This is the goal of the masters upon considering sex as a path by which one can reach spirituality and balance.

Through the practice of sex, woman may reach balance by taking from man the energy that she needs and vice versa. If men who practice Taoism must employ meditation and the conservation of semen and sexual energy, then women who practice Taoism (be they White Tigresses or not) must stimulate their sexual flows and energy.

This exchange is what allows men and women to obtain characteristics associated with the opposite sex: If woman is *Yin*, then she represents tranquility and receptiveness while man is *Yang* and represents activeness and creativity. Both sexes may take from their opposites, through sexual activity, the qualities they need to reach their maximum potential. For example, a plant needs water (*Yin*) and sun (*Yang*) to grow. If there is too much water, the plant dies; if there is too much sun, the same happens. A plant that grows with an abundance of sun will need more water to live. And so women, predominantly *Yin*, need masculine energy to flourish and the same goes for men and feminine energy.

If for Taoist men it is recommendable not to waste their energy on one or two women, for the Taoist women it is ideal to take from men, through seduction, the energy they need. The White Tigress seduces the Green Dragons to acquire energy and may live alongside a Jade Dragon when she finds it convenient, and she becomes its benefactor and protector. The relationship between the two is seen as mutual assistance in Taoist practices. These relationships tend to last two or three years.

There are no set rules for treating Dragons. A woman *tigress* may use exhibitionism to encourage them but also to feel her own sexual power. In order to extract from men the greatest amount of sexual energy, she uses submission and obsequiousness, which also pleases and benefits men in their own way. It is said that this type of woman tends to get down on her knees before the man (he on his knees or standing) to stroke and masturbate him or even to practice fellatio, since it is known that in general this is very pleasing for him and this posture tends to be very stimulating.

Long hair, wide hips, full red lips, long nails painted red, and a shaved Mound of Venus—female tigresses seduce men thanks to their appearance, which emphasizes their femininity. It is also, above all, a symbol of their power and success and of their desire to stay young.

Additionally, upon completing their education the Tigresses receive three emblems from their teacher: a tall choker that represents the collar of a domesticated tigress, a waist chain with a vial of jade that imitates the tooth of a tiger that contains a pearl of coagulated essence for good fortune, and a small tattoo on their Mound of Venus that increases their power.

The relationships between Tigresses and Dragons

"Where the Green Dragon must retain, the White Tigress must absorb. Where the Green Dragon seeks tranquility, the White Tigress seeks activity. Where the Green Dragon must be passive, the White Tigress must be aggressive. Like the two fish of Tai Chi, each one must seek its opposite to be complete."

The five essential activities

Since ancient times, man has felt the need to observe nature. The stars, the sun, and the moon have awakened their admiration and have led them to invent sophisticated apparatuses that allow them to see the universe more closely. Their curiosity has been without limit, and in their incessant quest to understand the energy that moves the world, the oriental wise men discovered that natural phenomena may be gradually understood. The conclusion is that each cycle may be divided in phases:

- **Water-winter-kidneys.** The energy is found at rest in states of stillness and extreme concentration like the seed of a tree or the reproductive cells of humans.

- **Wood-spring-liver.** The energy is active and begins to expand; this is a short period. As an example, we have the fertilization of the seed or the reproductive cells.

- **Fire-summer-heart.** During this prolonged period, the energy is released. This would be during the sprouting of the tree or the growth of the child.

- **Earth-Indian summer-spleen.** This is an inflection point and a time of balance during which the energy reaches the height of its expansion. It is the moment of maturity.

- **Metal-autumn-lungs.** The energy contracts. For example, the falling of the leaves or old age.

Life

All living things have *Yin* and *Yang* energies, and in their relationship with the world there is a constant flow of this energy, which differentiates them from inert beings. The Three Treasures make up part of life; they are the life within itself and they cannot be separated.

- **The *Jing* or vital essence.** It is made up of bodily fluids or moods (blood, lymph, semen, etc.). Natural immunological factors that allow for resistance to illnesses are located inside the *Jing*, which is, in fact, the base of vital activities.

  There are various types of *Jing*: the congenital, the acquired, that of the *Zang Fu* organs, and that of reproduction. These four *Jing* interact and change one another.

  The *Qi gong* exercises (known in ancient times as *Daoyin* or *Tao Yin*) are used to train, feed, and conserve *Jing* and to exercise the vital energy contained within the kidneys. The exercises and the conservation of sexual potency are useful for increasing the absorption of nutritional elements and strengthening the acquired *Jing*.

- **The *Qi, Chi,* or vital energy.** We are all born with an amount of *Qi* originating from our progenitors that with time diminishes. Lost *Qi* is recovered through the intake of food and water (energy from the earth), by breathing (energy from the sky), and through the exchange of fluids during the sexual act. Because of this, it is essential for good health to consume a proper diet, to breathe well, and to have an adequate sense of sexuality.

  Qi is the essential substance from which the world was formed. Every form of life requires *Qi*. Life is the fusion of *Qi*, death, and dispersion. *Qi* and *Jing* coexist and neither can exist without the other.

  Qi is stored in the kidneys and circulates through the whole body thanks to the labors of the heart, the lungs, the digestive process, and the stomach. *Qi* protects against illness, activates the circulation of blood, and maintains the temperature of an organism.

- **The *Shen* or spiritual body.** It is comprised of everything that allows us to interact with our surroundings: soul of the animal

(*Bo*), soul of the human (*Hun*), thought, intuition and conscience (*Yi*), and will (*Jir*). *Shen* relies on *Qi* and the existence of a corporal form in order to manifest.

Shen that is acquired (*Shishen*) is related to mental activity and is created through contact with nature after birth. The congenital or primordial *Shen* (*Yuanshen*) is the product of the combination of the masculine and feminine essences of the progenitors and controls vital activity. It is not controlled by mental activity, but both types of *Shen* must work together.

By living within society, a very complex and tiring environment, human beings suffer the anguish of the seven emotional factors and the six desires and often must resort to using the acquired *Shen* in an unbalanced way. The *Qi Gong* exercises are used to implant inner peace, thereby exiling the perverse thoughts and ideas that lead to the abuse of the acquired *Shen*.

The Three Treasures are not independent parts of a whole. Rather, they are three different manifestations of the one same reality that is life, where each treasure represents one aspect.

With an example, this concept of life will become clear. If we take three photographs of one object from different perspectives, we will have three distinct images. Each one shows the object differently, but none shows the object in its entirety nor are any of the images the object itself. *Jing*, *Qi*, and *Shen* are three manifestations of life, but none of them are life in its totality. None exists by itself.

The Three Treasures are interrelated because deep down they are all the same. Every alteration of one leads to alterations in the others. A sickness of the *Qi* will also be present in the entire living being, and when it develops fully, it will also be detected in the *Jing* and the *Shen*. Therefore, it is necessary to cultivate all three treasures in order to obtain good health. Thus, longevity depends upon the care of these three substances.

The meridians of energy

The meridians are invisible channels that are found in the interior of the body through which *Qi* flows. They function as a system different from the circulatory, nervous, and lymphatic.

Through the meridians, *Qi* is able to reach all of the tissues and organs of the body. It takes twenty-four hours for the energy to make the full journey through the web of channels.

There are two principal meridians, each one associated with one vital organ or function, and a number of minor channels.

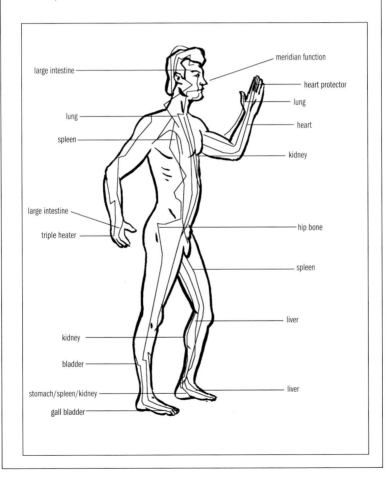

The concept of health and sickness

In a healthy individual, *Qi* is allowed to flow freely. When there is an excess of energy in one zone of the organism, according to the principle of self-regulation, the surplus energy flows toward the part of the organism that needs it or it exits the body spontaneously.

An organ that absorbs energy (concentration, *Yin*), upon having an excess, expels it spontaneously (expansion, *Yang*). When there is an excess of *Yin*, it suddenly becomes *Yang* and vice versa.

The *Yin-Yang* transformations allow for the self-regulation of the body and the maintenance of balance. But, given that these transformations depend on the flow of energy through the meridians, any obstacle in these channels will create excesses or shortages of energy in organs and tissues. When this happens, sickness is born. For this reason, Chinese medicine seeks to unblock the meridians through techniques such as massage, acupuncture, shiatsu, and breathing and physical exercises. It uses non aggressive techniques that reinstate the flow of energy, the effects of which can be seen at all levels.

Health through sex

If a man performs the act of sex just once without releasing semen, his vital essence is strengthened. If he does it two times, his sight and hearing sharpen. If he does it three times, all of his bodily illnesses disappear. If he does it four times, his blood circulation is reasonably improved. If he does it six times, his back becomes very strong. If he does it seven times, his thighs and gluteal muscles increase in strength. If he does it eight times, his whole body becomes resplendent and radiates. If he does it nine times, his life expectancy increases.

Yi-Fang; Pi-Chuch

Learning how to absorb sexual energy

White Tigresses know how to "absorb the breath of the Dragon," that is to say take advantage of the sexual energy of their lovers. This allows them to capture both mentally and physically the energy of the male organism and to use this energy (*Yang*) to complement and strengthen their own feminine energy (*Yin*). During this practice, tigress women must brighten their minds, which in this case is the experience of seeing many small lights moving in harmony inside their heads. They seek to use this experience of illumination nine times during different sexual encounters to produce enough energy to create their spiritual fetus of immortality.

A woman may use this illumination without having to circulate *Qi* through the meridians because she is spiritually and biologically ready for the pregnancy. For men, this is a much harder objective to reach, as they are not naturally ready for it. They may reach it through practices that revert *Ching* back to the brain, through the retention of sperm, and through meditation and breathing exercises. In any case, it is also hard for Tigresses to achieve nine separate illuminations in three years, and very few of them are able to.

The objective of their spiritual pregnancy is to exchange their mortal body for an immortal one. In order to progress, the Tigress must achieve the nine illuminations within the first three years of their training. These three years would correspond, when compared to the cycle of the Lepidoptera, to the formation of the larva, during which they dedicate themselves to refining the *Ching*, the sexual energy.

The next three years (the period of preservation) corresponds to the larva encasing itself in a chrysalis. During this, they concentrate on gathering *Qi*, vital energy, while the three years after that (the period of refinement) would end with the emergence of the perfectly formed butterfly. During this time they are almost dedicated to refining the *Shen*, the spirit and the conscience.

White Tigresses learn to conserve their youth by maintaining their bodies in puberty, as it is menstruation that causes unwanted changes and aging. Through a diverse number of exercises and care, they decrease their menstrual flow and their bodies remain vigorous and young.

- Massage exercises, which include techniques for self-massage, as well as massaging others.
- Specific *Kung Fu* techniques.
- Methods for restoration, such as shaving the pubis, inner cleansings, Ben Wa balls, chest massages, and exercises for tightening the vagina and strengthening the ovaries.
- Diets that manage weight, nourish the blood, and purify the body.
- Plants that regulate the menstrual flow and reinforce the immune system.
- Yoga exercises, willow waist exercises (see page 28), and back exercises.
- Transformation exercises, such as freezing the Jade Dragon, absorbing the breath of the Dragon, illumination, medicines of the three peaks, and immersion into orgasm.

Period of restoration. During this stage, tigress women must restore their youth completely and use absorption. The ideal age during which to initiate is 13 to 15 years old, as it is the time during which the woman still possesses the characteristics of adolescence that she wishes to keep throughout her whole life. The main objective is to completely restore the *Ching*.

This is what is learned during this stage:

- The ability to practice all the restoration exercises.
- How to decrease the menstrual flow.
- Prowess in all kinds of sexual stimulation.
- Familiarity with the transformation techniques.
- How to focus on absorbing the Dragon's breath and use the illumination of the mind on nine occasions.

Period of preservation. During these three years, tigress women concentrate on maintaining their youth and moving forward with absorption. Traditionally, they were able to adopt a disciple and gain independence from their teacher. In the past, many of them would become concubines, consorts, or courtesans in order to evolve while under the protection of a man and completely develop their *Qi* and *Ching*.

This is what is learned during this stage:

■ Mastery of the transformation techniques.
■ How to maintain a complete program of restoration exercises.
■ Beginning to teach other future tigress women.

Period of refinement. These are the final three years of learning. During this time, a tigress woman acts of her own accord and decides herself what she needs to progress. It is the stage of contemplative philosophy during which she joins her body (*Ching*), her breathing (*Qi*), and her spirit (*Shen*).

This new initiate only practices restoration exercises and transformation techniques that she deems necessary to perfect her immortality. She may have one Jade Dragon or various Green Dragons (that she no longer needs), or she may teach other women. She may also marry a man to whom she will never speak her secrets as a tigress woman unless he is an ancient Jade Dragon.

Basic exercises for a healthy life

Breathing exercises. When performed on a daily basis, these promote excellent health:

■ **Pectoral breathing.** This is what we normally use. It uses only the upper parts of the lungs. The thoracic cage opens and closes laterally, and the abdomen remains contracted during the whole process. This kind of breathing contributes to an increase in stress, anxiety, and hypertension.

■ **Abdominal breathing.** This consists of breathing by using the entire capacity of the lungs while relaxing the abdomen. This kind of breathing has a number of advantages: it favors blood and *Qi* circulation (energy of the body), massages the internal organs, relieves constipation caused by tension in the abdomen, and helps maintain inner calm and tranquility.

Abdominal breathing must be relaxed without forcibly inhaling or exhaling, and there must be no clear separation between one action and the next. The breathing must be fluid and without interruption. It is based on two movements:

1. **Inhaling.** Upon inhaling, the diaphragm (a membrane made of muscle fibers that separates the thoracic cavity from the abdominal cavity) dilates, which causes downward pressure, and the abdomen outwardly expands. It is advisable to contract the anal muscles in order to avoid losing any *Qi* that the body has gathered.

2. **Exhaling.** Upon expelling the air, the diaphragm exerts downward pressure, the abdomen contracts, and the anal muscles relax.

   If you are used to pectoral breathing, it is possible that you will be unable to learn the abdominal breathing technique simply by reading this lesson. This simple exercise will help you understand the process. Lie down face up and relax. Place a heavy book on the lower part of your abdomen (under the belly button). Inhale slowly and deeply through your nose and exhale calmly through your mouth. You will see that when you inhale, the book rises, and when you exhale, it falls.

   In this same way, when you are standing your abdomen expands when you breathe in and contracts when you exhale.

You must practice abdominal breathing when you wake in the morning, as you go to sleep at night, and before any stressful situation.

Different types of curative breathing

Tao advises several forms of breathing that are useful for specific situations:

- **Natural deep breathing.** Whenever there is fresh air and open space, one automatically breathes deeply, regardless of whether they are at the top of a mountain or the shore next to the sea. It is an action that revitalizes the entire being.

- **Cleansing breathing.** Inhaling through the nose and exhaling through the mouth. Releasing the air requires more time than inhaling it. It is useful for relieving inner tension or lowering a fever. The sigh is a spontaneous manifestation of this type of breathing.

- **Invigorating breathing.** Inhaling through the mouth and exhaling through the nose. The inhale is longer than the exhale. This method is used for gathering energy and increasing blood flow. Invigorating breathing is appropriate when lifting heavy objects or when preparing to plunge into a swimming pool.

- **Alternating breathing.** Inhaling through one nostril and exhaling through the other. This technique can be learned by practicing with the index fingers in the same way as with pranayama, a technique used in yoga. The right index finger closes the right nostril while air is inhaled through the left. Then the left index finger closes the left nostril as the air is exhaled through the right. Further along, it is possible to do this without the aid of fingers. With practice, breathing becomes long, slow, and deep. This technique may be used to relieve headaches and alleviate dizziness and worrying.

Good posture. Bad posture can cause skeletal deformities, a shortage of *Qi* circulation, and excessive pressure on the internal organs. In order to avoid illness, it is necessary to become conscious of the body and to relearn how to maintain good posture.

A correct body posture may be achieved using the first position of *Tai Chi*, the *Wu Chi* posture:

1. Stand up and feel how the soles of your feet are in contact with the ground. Distribute the weight of your body equally between

both feet. If the weight is balanced, there should be no tension in the waist.

2. Relax your shoulders, and let your shoulder blades remain gently curved; don't stretch your shoulders back nor your chest forward.

3. Imagine that a force is stretching you upward toward your crown. You will notice how the base of your skull gently lifts and your chin retracts. Don't lower your head, and keep staring forward. As you feel the stretch, concentrate your mind on your lower dantian, or the center of gravity of the body (the lower part of the torso located between the belly button and the pubis).

In this position, the axis of gravity of the body is perpendicular to the ground and the point of balance travels from the crown of the head to the feet and passes through the perineum. The body's weight is spread out through all the points, the head is not bent, the hands are hanging at the same height, and both feet are holding the same amount of weight.

A good body posture allows the body's center of gravity to stay within the dantian and produces an enjoyable feeling of balance and stability. Keep in mind that there is a direct correlation between posture and mood. A curved posture does not let energy flow and produces pressure in the heart, depression, and hypertension. On the other hand, a good posture allows for the circulation of energy and stimulates attentiveness and emotional balance.

Taoist exercises for women

The following exercises are used for strengthening and developing the breasts, decreasing menstrual flow, increasing the sensitivity of the nipples, and preventing tumors from forming in the chest.

These exercises should be done twice a day for one hundred days and afterward once a day only during menstruation.

Recovering the breasts. Sit with your legs crossed and your back straight. Place a cushion under your bottom to raise it up so your legs can touch the ground. It is recommendable to remove all your clothes, but you may place a blanket over your shoulders for warmth.

In order to prevent the loss of any *Qi* through the vagina during this exercise, place one of your heels against the opening or, if you are not flexible enough, place a ball against the vagina and hold it there with your foot. The following exercises are designed to bolster the breasts and keep them healthy.

- **Rub your hands together** to warm them up, and place one on each breast so that the nipples lie between the index finger and the thumb. Feel how the warmth of the hands enters the breasts. Carefully rotate the breasts. Your left hand will rotate in a counterclockwise direction while the right rotates in a clockwise direction. After twenty-four rotations, change direction.

- **Rub your fingertips together** to warm them up, and massage your nipples and areolas while moving your breasts in the manner described above. Do forty-eight rotations.

- **Massage** your entire breasts with your fingertips, making small circular movements. Do forty-eight rotations.

- **Place your hands back** on your breasts so that the nipples are between the index finger and the thumb. Inhale and pull the nipple away from you a little bit. Exhale and let go. Repeat this twenty-four times.

- **Warm your hands again** by rubbing them together, and place them back on your breasts like in the previous exercise so that you can feel the warmth.

Quickly contract your vagina and anus thirty-six times. Immediately after, press your breasts together so that they stick out and push them upward. Repeat this thirty-six times. Press your breasts together thirty-six times while at the same time lifting them upward. These exercises are excellent for stimulating circulation.

Tensing the vagina. Remain sitting and extend your legs in front of you. Move your ankles toward and away from each other as you inhale. Point the large toes on your feet outward and hold your breath at the same time as you clench your anus. Exhale and relax your feet and legs. Repeat this twenty-four times. This exercise strengthens the vaginal muscles and increases sexual energy.

Purifying the ovaries. As you lie back down with your legs together, warm your hands up and place them so that your index fingers are resting on your clitoris and your thumbs are touching your belly button, forming a rhombus. Press down on your ovaries using your ring and pinky fingers, and clench your vaginal and anal muscles through twelve breaths.

Next, while leaving your hands in place, take twelve deep breaths. Inhale through the nose and exhale through the mouth.

Open your legs and warm your hands again. Place the outer edge of each hand on each side of your pubic mound and massage vigorously until you feel the warmth. Roll onto the right side of your body. Put your right hand under your head beneath the ear. Place your left palm on your vulva. Move your left ankle over the right and keep your knees slightly bent. Breathe naturally with your attention on the lower part of your abdomen for five or ten minutes.

Willow waist exercises. These exercises are an excellent form of *Qi Gong* and are used to make the waist much more flexible and slim. They stimulate the internal organs in such a way that the body revitalizes itself and regulates the kidneys and intestines, fortifies the vaginal muscles, and strengthens the back. The exercises must be done daily. Your hands must move in a circular pattern in harmony with your waist and your breathing.

Upon doing these exercises, you must remember that when your hands move to the left of your body, your right hip must move to the right, and when your hands move to the right of your body, your left hip must move to the left.

When you inhale, make sure that the lower part of your abdomen is expanding. When you exhale, the lower part of your abdomen must contract. Breathe naturally.

Starting position

- Place your legs together so that your heels are touching.

- Place your hands on either side of your body so your fingers are touching the outside of your thighs.

- Keep yourself straight with your shoulders back and your head straight.

- Keep your tongue stuck against your palate; this will cause your mouth to secrete saliva, which helps with weight loss. Slowly breathe through your nose.

- When you inhale, tighten your vaginal muscles and imagine your nipples and areolas swelling and getting larger. When you exhale, relax your vaginal muscles and imagine your nipples becoming longer.

- Take nine deep and complete breaths to relax and calm your body. During this exercise, you should feel like a tiger climbing or stealthily moving among the trees.

Moving the tail down

- **First circle.** Starting from the initial position, put your hands together palm to palm and raise them to your chest. Move your arms to your left until you reach your right shoulder, which will lower until it is pointing toward the ground. Your hands must be pointing to the right. Exhale while you raise your hands and arms to the right, making a circle over your head.

The palms of your hands will form an open angle with the floor, and your left forearm will be at the same height as your forehead and parallel to the ground. As you are moving your arms to the right, move your head in the same direction. Inhale when your arms and hands pass over your head, and exhale when you reach the final position.

Now trace a complete circle with your hands and arms above your head. When you finish the movement, your fingers should be pointing to the right. Inhale during the first half of the circle and exhale during the second.

Move your waist as described in the previous section.

■ **Second circle.** Make another circle with your hands and arms but this time to the left in the same way described by the previous exercise.

Now you must trace another circle, but this time make the movement with your waist wider. Raise your hands and arms up and to the right, and make a circle until you come back around to the left side. When you finish the exercise, your fingers should be pointing straight down and to the left. Your shoulders should be lined up at chest height. Inhale during the first half of the circle and exhale during the second.

■ **Third circle.** In this part you will try to make a circle with your arms and hands by moving them from the left to the right and tracing an S as they move down. Start making the S when you get halfway down your body. Don't forget to move your hips to the opposite side of your hands.

Inhale while you raise your hands, and exhale when you trace the S. Immediately after, make another circle with your hands and arms from the right side of your body to the left. Raise your hands over your head, and when you go down, start making an S when you arrive at the height of your chest. Inhale as you go up, and exhale as you go down.

When you finish the movement, your fingers should be pointing downward with your right palm facing out.

Moving the tail up

- **First circle.** Start the exercise by leaning forward and tracing a circle to your left with your hands and arms until you reach your right side. As you descend, make an S at the height of your chest, and keep going until you reach your initial position. Point your fingers to the left to finish the movement.

  The whole movement contains two complete breaths. Inhale during the first half of the circle, and exhale when your hands start descending. Take another breath during the first half of the S, and exhale as you finish it.

  Make a complete circle with your arms and hands, moving them to your left side. As you move downward, make the shape of a hook. Finish this first circle leaning slightly forward and with your hands pointing down.

- **Second circle.** Make a circle around your head with your hands and arms. During the descent, make an S starting at chest height, and lean forward when you get to the lower part of the S. Move back while tracing a wide circle.

  Inhale during the first half of the circle, and exhale when you lower your hands. Inhale again during the first half of the S, and exhale during the second half. Finally, inhale one more time when you move your hands to the left, and exhale when they rise above your head for the last circular motion. You should finish with your hands pointing toward the right at chest height.

- **Third circle.** Trace three complete circles with your hands and arms, first by taking them from the right to the left and following the circle until they are back on the right side. Make an inverted S starting at chest height and finishing at the knees. Following this, trace another S from the bottom and going up. Your fingers will be pointing straight up at the left side of your body. Your right forearm will be parallel to the ground, and your left shoulder will be away from your body at chest level.

  Inhale during the first half of the circle, and exhale when you bring your hands to the front of your body at neck level. Inhale during the first half of the inverted S and exhale during the second half. Inhale again during the first half of the S and exhale during the last part.

To finish the exercise, bring your hands and arms up by the left side of your body until they are above your head. Your legs and feet must stay together. Inhale while you raise your arms and then lower them while you exhale with your elbows bent until they reach chest height. Finally, lower your hands and arms until they are parallel to your body. This last movement also contains a complete breath. You may repeat this series of movements four times. When you finish these exercises, sit down on the ground with your back straight and legs crossed and relax. Smile inwardly and feel your youth. Allow the energy to flow freely throughout your body.

The following exercises must be done after the waist exercises. Don't use too much force, as these are difficult exercises that require flexibility. They provide the body the same benefits as the waist exercises but are more efficient. They were used as an introduction to the *Kung Fu* exercises of the Taoist tigress women.

In Chinese culture, maintaining a strong and flexible back is a sign of youthfulness. Do the exercises slowly and progress little by little. Normally the Tigresses dedicated about six months to completing them, and they achieved a greater degree of flexibility.

Total flexibility. The objective of this exercise is to allow you to arch yourself completely backward until your body is held up by your feet and the palms of your hands. It should also be possible to bend forward until your head is between your legs.

Separate your legs until they are about twice as far apart as the distance between your shoulders. Lean backward with your arms raised and stuck to your head. Try to bring your head far enough back that you can see behind your back. Don't force yourself; when you reach the most that you can stretch, bring your torso up a little bit to relax your body during the stretch. When you are able to stretch far enough to see behind yourself, place a table behind you and lower yourself until you are able to place your hands firmly upon it. Raise your torso a little bit so that the stretch is more comfortable.

As this position becomes more and more comfortable, try lowering little by little the height of the supporting object until you are able to place your hands on the ground.

- **Leaning forward.** Slightly separate your feet to about half the distance between your shoulders. Slowly lower your torso by bending at the waist. If necessary, grab the back of your knees with your hands to help push yourself. Keep going slowly.

  When you are capable of bringing your head to your knees, practice by putting your hands on your ankles until you are able to put your head between your legs.

  Finally, you should be able to lift your hands around the outside of your legs until they can take hold of your waist or bottom, and your head should stay stretched out toward the back of your legs.

Grabbing yourself with your own "claws." The goal of this exercise is to be able to completely bend yourself forward from a seated position, grab the soles of your feet with your hands, and place your head between your knees and calves. The second goal is to be able to bend completely backward with your legs bent and a hand on each foot.

- **Bending forward.** Lie down on your back on a comfortable surface with your legs together and your ankles touching. Raise your torso and lean forward, bending at the waist, as far as you can. Grab onto your legs just under the knees in order to stretch as far as possible. As you progress with this exercise, you will be able to hold onto your ankles in order to lower yourself. Finally, grab your feet and let your head rest between your knees and calves. It will take several months for you to successfully complete this exercise.

■ **Bending back.** Sit on the ground with your knees bent and your feet placed further apart than your thighs. Lean back gently, placing your hands behind you for support. Keep lowering yourself, and as you practice the exercise, you will be able to grab the lower part of your feet and, further on, stretch until you are completely stretched out.

Stretching the legs. The goal of this exercise is to be able to raise each leg in front of your body until they are close to your head.

Lay on your back on a comfortable surface. Put both hands behind one of your knees and gently push, with your knee bent, toward your chest. When you are able to place your knee on your chest, straighten your leg in order to accentuate the stretch. At first, you will not be able to stretch your knee all the way to your chest; straighten your leg as far as it will go, but do it gently. Later on, you will be able to place your leg next to your head.

Scratching the back part of your head. The point of this exercise is to be able to bring your ankles, together or separately, behind your neck.

Sit on a soft surface with your legs completely bent and your head touching the ground. Place one of your ankles behind your neck. Gradually sit up until you are sitting straight.

When you are able to do this with either leg, try raising the other.

Upon completing the exercises, feel how the youthfulness and energy flow through your veins.

The inner smile

The organs absorb, process, and store *Qi*, the energy of the body, and their good work deserves our thanks in the form of the inner smile. The inner smile consists of taking stock of our organs and including them in our perception of our bodies as a whole, thus allowing energy to flow through the body. This is a powerful and simple relaxation technique that tones and purifies the vital organs.

When any part of our body stops functioning correctly, we repudiate and try to ignore it while hoping that it will not infect the rest. We think that if we mentally isolate this one area, the pain will disappear. What is happening, however, is quite the opposite; we are restricting the flow of energy and making a path for the illness. We cannot fix our problems by shoving them in a corner because they will end up taking control of us without our even noticing.

The inner smile not only helps us change the inner state of our body, but it also teaches us to send positive energy through our organism and interact with it, which creates an inner state of harmony.

In Taoism, the consciousness reigns not only in the brain but throughout the whole body. And so, just like when we act unconsciously and suddenly become conscious thereby creating a sense of inward movement and vibration, the same happens with our vital organs. Once we begin to see our body as one interconnected whole, we may begin to interact with any part of it. In the same way that we say "me" and smile as we become conscious of ourselves, we can also say "my heart" or "my liver," for example, and feel them as we smile inwardly at them.

The inner smile, which helps to dissolve physical and mental stress, is used as a preparation or warm up for other types of meditation.

Inner smile exercises

- The aperture of fire of the heart, used for burning negativity and regenerating positivity, is the first level of practicing the inner smile. To begin the exercise, sit comfortably on the edge of a chair with your feet flat on the ground. Keep your back straight without straining it. Bring the palms of your hands together in your lap; your right palm will rest on top of your left.
- Close your eyes, and feel your connection to the ground through your feet. Bond with the energy of the earth.
- Become conscious of yourself sitting on the chair with your hands together. Place your tongue against your palate. Conjure up, about three feet in front of you, an image of your own self smiling or that of someone you love and respect.

➤

- Become conscious of the point between your eyebrows from which you are projecting this energy. Relax and open your Third Eye (*Ajna chakra*). Gather the energy of your smile between your eyebrows, and allow it to spread through your whole body.

- The energy of the smile will travel from the middle of your forehead while relaxing your cheeks, nose, mouth, and facial muscles. As it descends through your neck, gently rotate your head from side to side to relax it.

- Allow the energy to flow through the back of your sternum. This is where your thymus gland is, which governs the heart and the circulatory system and is known also as the house of the heart. Feel how it becomes warmer and starts to vibrate as it expands.

- Lift your palms, still together, and place your thumbs against the middle of your heart. Let the energy radiate from the thymus gland to the heart. Don't forget to continue creating more energy between your eyebrows and let it cascade downward through your body to your heart. Smile inwardly at your heart to renew its capacity for happiness. Do not move on until your heart is filled with loving energy. This way, you will disperse the negative energies of stress, cruelty, and arrogance.

- Pronounce the sound of the heart. As you exhale, say "Haaaaaoooo- ouu," and direct the breath toward your heart. The ember of love that you have created inside it will burn the negative feelings and keep the pure red essence of the heart. Feel how the heart becomes redder and stronger each time until it transforms into a precious ruby. Little by little, make it bloom like a great flower and leave behind any negative emotions, such as scorn, hate, arrogance, or resentment. Let the regenerative energy expand to the rest of your body.

- Remember the sensation that this exercise produces so you may recall it at any time during the day when you feel depressed, nervous, or unhappy. The more you feel it, the easier it will be to recall it.

- Conclude the exercise by collecting all the energy in your dantian (or *Tan Tien*) situated one and a half inches below your belly button on the inside of your body. This is where you store the *Qi* that you inherited from your parents. The inner smile helps blocked *Qi* to flow and creates new *Qi* that enriches what is already there.

- Smile at your belly button, and collect all the energy in the palms of your hands and move them in an outward spiral thirty-six times. Men must make this movement in a clockwise direction and women in a counterclockwise direction. Next, switch directions and turn the spiral inward.

Relaxation exercises

These exercises loosen up the joints and allow for a free flow of *Qi* through the whole body. This results in relaxation of the mind. Thanks to this, we will be in optimal condition for performing massage. These are very important exercises for staying in shape and are a great warm up for any aerobic or other muscle exercise.

During every exercise, your concentration must be on your lower dantian, which is the center of gravity of the human body. You must not force yourself; any pain indicates that you have gone beyond your limits and must be gentler. The motions must be done slowly and with concentration.

As you do these exercises, imagine that you have heavy metal balls on your hands and feet that require a great deal of tension and articulation in your muscles to allow movement. After doing these exercises, you will feel refreshed and relaxed.

Waist

1. Stand up in the *Wu Chi* position with your feet spread apart a little farther than the distance between your shoulders. Keep yourself straight and relax your shoulders. Stare fixedly but calmly at a single point at eye level.

2. Swing your hips back and forth from one side to the other. You should not move your shoulders or head. Keep looking straight ahead. You will notice that the movement of your hips is done using your waist muscles, not the muscles running from your shoulders to your back.

3. When you have swung your hips around about ten times, start moving them with more force. You will find that your arms are pulled along by the movement and that you are no longer moving just your hips but also the middle part of your torso and, eventually, the top part of your torso and neck. You will also notice that your knees and heels are rotating along your vertical

axis. You head should hardly move, and your gaze should stay firmly fixed on the same spot.

4. Rotate about forty times to each side.

Opening the Door of Life

1. Place yourself in the *Wu Chi* position. Swing your hips, chest, shoulders, neck, and head at the same time as one toward the left and slightly forward. Immediately after, raise your right arm to eye level, palm facing outward as if you were drawing a curtain. At the same time, bend your left arm and place the back of your hand behind your back on top of the Door of Life (the spot on your back at the same height as your belly button).

2. In this position, spin your hips to the left as far as they will go without straining. If you have done the exercise correctly, the part of your spine belonging to the Door of Life will stretch. If only your shoulders stretch, begin again. When you are able to stretch the Door of Life, relax and then stretch two more times. Then do the same exercise while turning to the right. You must turn nine times to each side and stretch three times for every turn.

Stretching the vertebrae between the sky and earth
FIRST SEQUENCE

1. We will begin with the *Wu Chi* position. Without raising your arms, place your hands in front of your body, palms inward, and hook your thumbs together. With your thumbs still together, raise your hands to shoulder height without raising your shoulders. Next, breathe in as you stretch your arms upward, as if you were touching the sky with your fingertips. Lean your head lightly back, and open your mouth as if to yawn.

2. Now start breathing out slowly and stretch forward while keeping your head between your arms, and bend your back bit by bit until you are touching the ground. Throughout the exercise, you will notice your vertebrae stretching beginning at the lower back and ending at the neck.

3. Straighten back up slowly without raising your arms, and as you do this, feel the weight of your head.
Now lift your arms as you did at the beginning of the exercise while reaching toward the sky.

4. Repeat this sequence four times.

SECOND SEQUENCE
During this exercise, your arms appear to push water over your head and behind you. This differs from the previous exercise, during which it appears you are gathering water toward your body.

1. Join your thumbs, and lift your elbows to shoulder height like in the previous exercise. Drag the palms of your hands down along your torso until your arms are extended, and start bending your back forward. Relax your neck muscles so your joints may stretch correctly.
2. With your body bent and your head between your arms, start to straighten up while bringing your arms forward and then up. While doing this, keep your head between your arms. At the end, your fingers will be pointing toward the sky and your head will be bent slightly back, like at the end of the previous exercise.
3. Repeat the second part of this sequence four more times.

THIRD SEQUENCE
While doing this exercise, you will take on the appearance of a windmill or a clock.

1. Place yourself in the final position of the previous exercises, that is to say with your arms stretched upward and your head between them. Twist your torso, arms, and head as a whole toward the left without moving your hips. You will notice the right side of your waist stretching.

Lower your torso with your arms and head downward and toward the left. As you lower, turn little by little to the right until you are completely bent with your hands in front of your feet. Keep turning to the right as you lift your chest, arms, and head. When you reach the same posture as at the beginning of the exercise, you have finished.

2. Repeat this rotation four times.

3. Now you must repeat the sequence in the opposite direction beginning with a stretch to the right. You must also do this four times.

Shaking out. This will most likely be the simplest part of these exercises for you. You must first restore balance to your body and relax it completely. Get rid of all your inner tension through the movement.

1. Stand up with your feet apart and your arms crossed. Shake your whole body by rapidly bending and stretching your knees and keeping your muscles relaxed. Your whole body will be affected by the movement, and you will feel the shaking in your bottom, chest, etc. It feels just like riding a train without tensing your muscles. If it is hard to rapidly shake out your body, try adding some music to the exercise. Do this for a whole minute.

2. Women must complement the upward and downward shakes with additional lateral shaking. Rotate your hips in a circle around your body's vertical axis while switching directions intermittently. Every change in direction must be accompanied by a strong jerk of the hip in the direction of the last circle. Make about ten circles in each direction. Next, rapidly shake your hips and shoulders laterally, similar to how you were shaking to the front at the beginning of the exercise. Do this for a whole minute.

3. Now, men as well as women must finish with the most entertaining part of the exercise: kicks and whip lashes. Kick three times to the front, three times to the side, and three times to the back with each leg. Now imagine that you are holding a whip and crack it three times in each of the three directions previously indicated with each hand. If you add a high-pitched shout with each movement, you will feel like new.

All these individual exercises are thought not only to increase flexibility but to also get fully in the mood when performing erotic massage.

Having a full sense of sexuality contributes to the corporal and spiritual balance of the couple. When we make love, we don't leave just leave our clothes behind in order to feel closer to the other person, but we also do it to leave behind our stress and problems so that our energy may flow in harmony.

The spirituality of the sexual act in which body and soul melt together is reached by starting with an adequate physical and mental disposition. Breathing, having a positive attitude, relaxation, etc. are all things that should not be ignored in order to achieve complete pleasure.

Let your energy flow normally through all the channels of your being so that *Yin* and *Yang* may be in complete balance and project serenity and desire to your partner.

Sexuality according to Taoism

Upon looking, we do not see it, as it is invisible.
Upon listening, we do not hear it, as it is inaudible.
Upon touching it, we do not feel it, as it is impalpable.
These three qualities (invisible, inaudible, impalpable)
make up the Self.

Sexual energy, *Ching Chi* or *Jing Chi*, is a form of *Qi*, the vital energy. Part of this sexual energy is passed down from our parents and may become lost if we do not replenish it. When this energy completely fades away, we die.

Taoism teaches us how to collect more energy through sex and gathering aspects from our sexual partner that complement us. If men who observe the *Tao* must hold themselves back in order to absorb the *Yin* of women, then White Tigresses must learn to extract the *Yang* energy that they need from their Green Dragons in specific ways, among them fellatio. To a White Tigress, coitus is not the most effective way of obtaining energy, although she may still employ it with moderation.

The importance of sexuality

As we saw in chapter one, the Three Treasures are able to morph into one another in the same way that energy can morph into substance (for example, when we absorb *Qi* of the earth through food and transform it internally into tissue, which is *Jing*, or substance), spirit into energy, etc. The sexual act is one of the moments during which this transformation happens.

Sexuality is of great importance to Taoism; it is considered a source of health and spiritual growth. During sex, there is a great buildup of *Qi*, or energy of the body, that explodes during orgasm. During this explosion, *Qi* energy becomes *Jing* (substance) and *Shen* (spirit) energy.

In fact, the customs of Taoism aim to keep the energy that is hatched during orgasm from escaping the body so that it may be transformed into *Jing* and *Shen* to the benefit of oneself and the couple.

During orgasm, *Qi* energy turns into a number of other substances: semen in the man and vaginal, salivary, and mammary secretions in the woman. These substances possess immunological properties and are very nutritional and, therefore, must not be wasted. Men possess the ability to control ejaculation, and women may swallow their own saliva, as well as making use of the man's semen for curative and rejuvenating purposes. Women also tend to reabsorb substances during the sexual act, meaning that there is generally not a great loss of energy.

Qi that accumulates during orgasm is also transformed into *Shen* when the energy is made to rise from the lower dantian, or the sexual core, upward through the spine. This is why the act of sex is considered to be of benefit to inner peace and clarity of the mind.

Man and woman

The fundamental difference between men and women lies in their sexual tolerance. Men, by nature, lose energy during sex upon discharging semen to the outside, while women automatically reabsorb their secretions and do not tire. Given the content of energy and the curative power of these fluids, men must compensate for said loss through certain Taoist practices that will be explained in the following section. Women lose their energy during menstruation, thus they must also resort to Taoist customs to replenish it.

Another difference between the sexes is that men show a faster sexual reaction when faced with exterior stimulation than women do, meaning that they must learn to control their reactions at will. If the man initiates sex before the woman is prepared, he will reach orgasm before she does, which sparks devastating consequences for both. If the man ejaculates without first absorbing the fluids secreted by the woman during orgasm, he will suffer a great loss of energy. For this reason, Taoism instructs the man to observe the woman's sexual attitude, respond accordingly, and avoid premature ejaculation by controlling it. On the other hand, Taoism also teaches to separate orgasm and ejaculation.

To a woman who practices Taoism, sex is much more than a man entering and exiting her vagina. She continues conceptualizing sex with the same emotion as in her adolescence but with greater knowledge. She does not have sex in order to satisfy her urgent needs but to enjoy the romance, the emotion, and the adventure. It is not penetration in and of itself that rejuvenates but everything that sex involves: fantasizing, stroking, touching, dressing, tasting, showing, watching, kissing, playing, inventing... A White Tigress is conscious of the need to recreate the curiosity, intensity, and emotion of her first sexual encounters in order to enjoy the full benefits of sex.

The sexual philosophy of the tigress woman

The Portal of the Sky (mouth), when used sexually, stimulates the Shen (mind/ spirit) and may have spiritual benefits.

The Jade Door Opening (vagina), when used sexually, tends to stimulate the Ching (sexual/bodily energy) and has physical effects.

Exchanging energy during the act of sex

The substances that a woman secretes during sex must be absorbed by the man in order to compensate for his loss of energy. Let us read an excerpt from the writings of Wu Hsien, a follower of Taoism from the 1st century B.C.

> The highest peak is called the "Red Lotus Peak." Its essence is "The Jade Spring," and flows from two conduits beneath the woman's tongue, and is transparent with a neutral flavor. The man must lap up these secretions with his tongue and swallow them, as they are exceedingly beneficial to one's health. This medicine boosts the functions of the five internal organs, nourishes intuition, provides *Qi*, and strengthens the blood.

As far as tigress women are concerned, tradition dictates that they must learn to store their saliva and combine it with the rain of the Dragon (the fluid preceding ejaculation) that, when mixed with the woman's saliva, produces the Great Medicine. Swallowing this mixture during orgasm delays the aging process in the woman. According to Wu Hsien:

> The middle peak takes the name of "Twin Peaks." Its essence is called "White Snow" and is secreted by the woman's nipples. Its color is white and it tastes slightly sweet. Of the three libations, this one is, without doubt, superior, especially if the woman has not breastfed before. Upon drinking it, the man fuels his core (spleen and stomach), tones his whole body, and grows his *Shen* (spirit). A woman who allows the drinking of this medicine experiences an improvement to the circulation of her blood.

According to this tradition, women must drink this fluid of their own accord, although they would not be able to do so without help unless they are able to reach their own nipples or are bisexual. Tigresses must ask a man to conserve this medicine in their mouths and then take it from him. And the last libation:

> The lower peak receives the name "Dark Portal." Its essence is the "Lunar Flower" and lies in the deepest parts of the *Yin*

Palace (upper part of the vagina). This liquid is very lubricating. However, the *Yin* Palace is nearly always closed, and opens only when the woman is aroused to the point at which her face reddens and her voice becomes a moan. It is then that the essence flows. If a man wishes to drink this liquid, he must withdraw his *Yang* Shield (penis) until he is barely penetrating the woman's cavern. This will fortify his primordial *Yang* (sexual force). Such are the Libations of the Three Peaks.

According to advanced traditional practice, women may ingest this elixir after their own orgasm or, sometimes, place it on the head of the man's penis and mix it with her own saliva and the rain of the Dragon. This secretion will rejuvenate her. She may also recharge her energy reserves with her own saliva that is produced upon arousal or the act of oral sex and also with semen.

One must keep in mind that, according to proponents of acts of oral sex, saliva is a bodily fluid that contains many nutrients that benefit the body; it is considered, for example, of benefit to digestion. Salivating in abundance may aid with weight loss and heal the skin, teeth, and gums, as well as cleaning the esophagus. In Taoism, saliva is also called divide water or juice of jade and is valued because, upon ingestion, it rejuvenates, cleans, and regenerates the body. For Taoists, it is a key ingredient for good health and for creating the Elixir of Immortality.

In this sense, semen is a bodily fluid containing proteins that helps to create fresh blood in the part of the body upon which it is applied. However, in the same way that the Chinese tigress woman does not use a Green Dragon more than nine times, one must remember that no modern woman should take risks. Following this, it is important to avoid men who ejaculate inside. Applying semen to the body keeps the skin and hair healthy.

In order to prevent sexually transmitted diseases and aid in the revitalization of the body and blood, later generations take one aspirin every day. Recent studies have shown that the coverings used in many medications, aspirin among them, defend against STDs. In any case, tigress women never take risks.

Complementary youth treatments

■ **Steam baths.** These are very effective at purging the body of toxins, stimulating blood flow, and increasing the size of the breasts and nipples, which during the bath will be covered by a tightly rolled towel.

While taking a steam bath, the woman must be seated with her legs open and her right index finger inserted in her vagina up to the knuckle. She should contract her vagina and anus thirty-six times. When her body starts to sweat, she will rotate her breasts thirty-six times in one direction and thirty-six times in the opposite direction, as explained in the section on curative exercises.

■ **Diet.** It is free of fats and lactose products and rich in protein. Beef is not eaten, as it is considered to be full of toxins. Other types of meats, soy products, or fish and shellfish may be eaten.

■ *Dong Quai.* Many of the exercises for initiates aim to decrease the menstrual flow and regulate menstruation. The *Dong Quai*, which should not be taken by pregnant women or women with asthma, regulates menstruation, decreases the flow, increases sexual energy and vitality, and augments the breasts. Taoist women drink one cup of *Dong Quai* tea every morning.

■ **Cleaning using a cucumber.** Once a week, except during menstruation, some women will take a small peeled cucumber and insert it in their vagina. To clean, she will rotate it. The cucumber is also a good cleanser for the mouth.

■ **Dragon pearls.** They are known as Chinese balls or Ben Wa (internal use) balls. They are inserted in the vagina for stimulation and have a smaller ball inside that produces a ringing noise like a bell. The best ones are made of jade.

Some tigresses leave them in their vaginas for at least six hours a day to stimulate sexual secretions, rejuvenate themselves, and avoid stress.

■ **The vertical.** Doing the vertical is a very useful exercise for women because it stimulates blood flow and prevents cold hands and feet. The exercise should last between five and ten minutes. Do this exercise close to a wall so you can support yourself and be more comfortable.

Stand 1.5 meters (about 5 feet) in front of the wall. Raise your arms above your head. Take a step forward and place your hands in front of you on the floor, shoulder-width apart, about 30 centimeters (almost 1 foot) from the wall. Using momentum, place yourself face down and kick your leg against the wall. Afterward, continue with the other leg. Keep your arms straight. Keep your legs straight and together. Squeeze your stomach and back so that it doesn't bend or flex the hip.

Start by remaining in this posture one minute each day during the first week, two minutes a day during the second, and three minutes a day during the third. During the fourth week, increase the time until you can endure ten minutes each day. After one hundred days of practicing, you will only need to do this exercise twice a week.

As an alternative to this, there are two yoga postures, over the shoulders (sarvangasana) and over the head (sirsasana).

■ **Freezing the Jade Dragon.** Tigress initiates can use this technique during the first three years of their apprenticeship (they would abandon it afterward). It is thought that by freezing the Jade Dragon, one can increase their capacity for absorbing the breath of the Dragon. To do this, the woman receives the semen of the Jade Dragon on her face and allows it to coagulate, which separates the seminal fluids from the sperm. On her knees, the Tigress waits for the moment of ejaculation and directs it toward her face. The Tigress is interested not only in the semen but also in the sexual energy given off by the man. This is why she pays close attention to the start of ejaculation and lets the man release himself so that he may enjoy the most of her before directing his penis toward her face.

At the end of a minute or however long it takes the sperm to coagulate, the Tigress rubs it over her face and lets it dry for three minutes.

Exercises for increasing sexual prowess

These exercises increase sexual stamina and increase the amount of pleasure. Both members of the couple can practice these.

Strengthening the core energy of the body. This exercise strengthens the Cinnabar Field, the energy core located at the height of the belly button, in which the transformation from *Jing* into *Qi* takes place and vice versa.

1. Sit on the ground with your legs together and knees straight. In this position, grab your feet with your hands so that your palms are touching the soles your feet and your arms are stretched out on either side of your calves.

2. Maintain this position for about a minute while breathing deeply.

Acupressure. In order to perform the following massages, you will need to locate the different areas on the body that you need to touch or apply pressure to with your hands. Treatment through shiatsu is discussed more in depth in the chapter about enjoying sex with acupressure (page 131).

The box on the following page shows two of the main areas needed to perform the suggested treatments. These may be applied before foreplay, as a part of the foreplay, combining them with a sensual massage, or by themselves, although their effectiveness is greater in the first case. It is important to persevere and not to trust only in shiatsu to solve problems or improve but to maintain an adequate frame of mind. Be receptive and continue to practice the other exercises detailed in this book, especially those that strengthen the love muscle.

Where to find them

	Point 1. Double point located on the sole of each foot. If you bend your toes and squeeze both sides of your feet, the point will be at the intersection of the resulting lines.
	Point 3. Located on the back of the hand between the metacarpal bones of the thumb and index finger.
	Point 7. This point is found on the abdomen just under the belly button. **Point 11.** Double point located on the belly button's vertical line.
	Point 14. Double point found above both knees, just over the kneecap, at the spot where the knee ends and the thigh begins.
	Point 16. Double point located under the knee between the two bones belonging to the lower leg, the tibia and the fibula.
	Point 17. Double point located above the ankle on the back of the tibia.
	Point 21. Double point found at the beginning of the second toe just a few fractions of an inch away from the toenail.
	Point 22. Double point located at the beginning of the back between the shoulder blades, specifically between the second and third vertebrae, on both sides of the spine.
	Points 27, 28, 29, and 30. Located on the lower back on the sacrococcygeal bone. They are one on top of the other.

There are about three hundred and sixty points on the human body, but in this book we will only deal with those having to do with sex and sexual energy.

Transferal of sexual energy between partners. This treatment allows for the transfer of sexual energy between both members of a pair. Whoever has the most sexual energy can give it to their lover if they are feeling weak. The person who wishes to receive the energy will stand in front of their partner. Using the middle finger of each hand, touch point 1, located on your partner's feet. The contact should be prolonged and without the application of pressure. It should also be done before initiating foreplay.

Pumping Energy

1. Locate double point 21 and apply pressure by pinching or softly squeezing the skin together for a minute.

2. Find point 7 and apply pressure in a circular motion just hard enough to move the skin in the same pattern for a minute.

3. Seek out double point 11 and apply the same type of pressure as before for the same amount of time.

4. Now look for double point 17 and apply considerable and constant pressure for half a minute. You must press down on the point with your thumb while holding tightly to the rest of the area with your hand. As long as you continue to apply pressure, you must retain contact between your fingers and the area you are treating. It is recommendable to combine pressure and distention to stimulate the pumping of energy.

5. Afterward, locate double point 22 and apply pressure with your thumb for one minute.

6. Finally, find double point 14 and apply pressure with your thumb for one minute.

Dynamizing sexual energy

1. Find double point 17 and apply pressure by holding tight.

2. Locate double points 27, 28, 29, and 30. Close your fist and place each one of your four knuckles on one of the points and apply pressure to all of them simultaneously. First, apply pressure to all the points on one side and then on the other side. Do this for two minutes on each side.

General Cleansing

1. Locate double point 3 and pinch, applying pressure for half a minute always in the direction of the second metacarpal while combining pressure and then letting up of pressure. Pressing this point alleviates headaches, toothaches, facial and menstrual pain, and constipation.

2. Immediately after, find double point 16 and apply pressure by holding tightly. This point bolsters the entire organism.

3. Locate double point 17 and apply pressure in the same manner as the last point.

Strengthening the lumbar area. The area we are treating is the lumbar (between the waist and coccyx), where the genital nerves are concentrated.

Apply light pressure for about five seconds, let up, and reapply pressure nine more times in order to strengthen these nerves.

For older men, applying gentle pressure to the testicles while complementing with soft strokes proves very effective.

Treating against inhibition. Start by applying circular pressure to double point 1 for three or four minutes. Follow up with a vigorous and passionate massage. This method eases fear of sexual relationships and is used to treat cystitis, dysmenorrhea, and urinary incontinence. It also bolsters the sex organs and immune system.

How to massage

METHOD	TECHNIQUE
Pressure by pinching	Softly pinch the area you wish to treat between your thumb and index finger.
Circular pressure	Rotate the skin with your index and middle fingers while applying light pressure. You may also use the tips of all your fingers.
Pressure by gripping	Exert pressure on the area to be treated using your thumb, and keep the skin in contact with the rest of your hand. Activate your energy.

Opening your small circulation. Meditation of the Microcosmic Orbit is a meditative technique that improves the flow of Qi through the small circulation, a circle formed by the governing vessel (through which Qi ascends through the back of the body from the bottom of the spine to the spot between your eyebrows while passing through the crown) and by the functional vessel or glass of conception (through which Qi descends through the front of the body and from the space between your eyebrows to the Cinnabar Field, also called the lower dantian).

As previously mentioned, the Three Treasures, *Jing* or substance, Qi or energy, and *Shen* or spirit, may transform into each other. So *Shen* may become Qi through meditation. Spiritual concentration (*Shen*) allows for an increase in sexual energy (Qi).

When the mind concentrates on one part of the body, it is capable of causing energy to flow to it. This idea is explained in classic Taoist texts thusly, "The mind directs and Qi follows." This exercise will cause the energy that is spread throughout the entire body to concentrate on the dantian in the form of sexual energy and flow through the small circulation while passing through different gates and energy cores along the way.

Within the body there exist the following energy cores or gates: the dantian, the perineum (the area between the anus and the genitals), the coccyx (at the end of the spine), the Ming Men or Gate of Life (under the second vertebra of the lumbar between the kidneys and behind the belly button), the crown, the space between the eyebrows or the Third Eye, the spot between the breasts (point 40), and the palms of the hands and soles of the feet. Through these gates we may, using meditation, absorb the Qi of our surroundings and expel used Qi. In this manner, passing through each gate increases the quantity and quality of sexual energy in the body.

Once we abandon meditation, the sexual energy that flowed through the small circulation spreads back throughout the body along every meridian, increasing the overall energy.

Perform the following meditations to open the small circulation. Keep in mind that mastery of this exercise requires a great deal of practice.

1. Sit on the floor with your legs crossed, your hands on your knees, and your back straight while looking ahead.

2. Close your eyes and breathe deeply. When your breathing becomes fluid and quiet, start breathing abdominally (see page 24) and focus all your attention on the lower dantian. As you breathe deeply, you will feel your dantian becoming warmer and filling with sexual energy. You will feel slight vibrations in this area. Primordial Qi, your sexual energy, is accumulating in your lower dantian. When the vibrations become more noticeable, begin moving the energy along your small circulation.

3. First, concentrate on the belly button and try to compress the energy even more. Proceed to the sexual core (Palace of the Sperm or Ovaries), located where the prostate or ovaries are found. Next, concentrate on the perineum.
To conduct the energy from one spot to another, one uses light general meditation, and to pass through one of the gates, one uses deep concentrated meditation. During both of these types of meditation, the mind must be blank and devoid of any concrete thought.

4. When you have passed through the gate at the perineum and feel the heat, pain, or tingling in this area (an unmistakable sign

that the *Qi* energy has rekindled), proceed toward the coccyx. Next, direct your energy upward, increasing in intensity through your spine, passing through the Gate of Life (the point on the backbone between the lower neck and shoulder blades), and through the crown. End at the spot between your eyebrows, thus finishing the journey through the governing vessel.

5. You must now connect the functional vessel with the governing vessel. To do this, concentrate on the tip of your tongue and press it against your palate. Apply and relieve pressure about twenty-five times. Afterward, focus your mind on the point located in the center between the breasts and feel how the energy descends toward it. Travel through this gate, and proceed along the descent toward the dantian, thereby completing the circle.

You must start by completing about ten cycles and will increase that number as you gain more experience. If during this exercise you begin to feel your energy flowing freely, do not try to hinder it.

The post

This exercise stretches the muscles and tendons that unite the thighs and pelvis and bolsters the flow of *Qi* through the meridians that travel from the feet to the perineum, as well as increasing sexual potency. Repeat this exercise three times.

1. Stand up and place your legs apart. Open your feet so that the toes on both feet are pointing in opposite directions. Extend your pelvis forward, tightening your buttocks, and place your hands on your thighs.

2. Keep your back straight and without relaxing your buttocks lower your chest by bending your knees and opening your pelvis. This position will feel strained, but try to hold it for as long as you can. Afterward, lightly kick the air a few times to relax the thigh muscles.

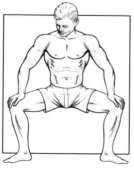

Exercise of the Buddhist monk. These exercises will be done while sitting on the ground. They are used to strengthen the lower abdominal muscles, which play a part in controlling the clitoris and the erection of the penis.

1. Sit on the ground with your legs crossed and place your hands on your knees. Keep your back straight and stare ahead during the whole exercise.

2. Lean forward about 45 degrees and then straighten back up. Lean back as far as possible. Straighten back up again. You should not be bending your head forward or backward; it should remain in line with your chest during the entire exercise.

3. Repeat this as many times as you can (at least twenty) until you are tired, and do the entire sequence about ten times a day.

Toning exercise. This exercise strengthens the abdominal muscle and improves sexual potency, as well as improving the flexibility and strength of the waist muscles.

It may be that at the beginning, you have a little trouble completing the exercise, as it requires some effort to do the stretches. However, with practice the amount of effort required will decrease, and you will notice that you are much more flexible. Those who suffer from arteriosclerosis or hypertension should not do this exercise.

1. Lie down on the ground and raise your legs by about 20 degrees. Place the palms of your hands on the ground to keep from sliding forward.

2. Without bending your knees, alternately raise your right leg while lowering the left and vice versa without letting them touch the ground. Do this about thirty times. Rest your legs on the ground.

3. Next, bring both legs together and raise them by about 90 degrees. Slowly point your legs, without bending or splitting them, to the left as you lower them. Lift them back up by 90 degrees, and lower them now toward the right. Do this ten times in each direction.

4. Stay spread out and bend your knees with the bottoms of your feet on the ground. Place your hands on your stomach and raise the upper part of your body and your head as one whole without bending your neck. You will notice your abdominal muscles at stomach height compressing. Repeat this exercise twenty times.

5. Lie face down on the ground with your legs straight and slightly apart and your hands crossed behind your neck. Lift your chest and legs at the same time about fifteen times.

Exercises for men

URINATING ON TIP TOES

This exercise is very beneficial for men. The strength of the flow of urine is indicative of sexual prowess. A strong flow means a lot of sexual energy, and a weak and interrupted flow means very little. As a result, it is important to care for the health of the kidneys and to stimulate them when practicing the number of exercises for increasing sexual potency.

This exercise develops the muscle that is used during urination and the act of sex. It will help achieve a stronger flow of urine and increase sexual potency.

The technique consists simply of forcing the flow of urine, standing on tip toes, and gritting your teeth. Remember this beneficial exercise every time you relieve yourself.

ABSORBING SUN RAYS

The best time to do this exercise is at sunrise, and the best season is during spring. It is best to do it while naked. You must stand before the sun and breathe deeply. The sun's energy will gather in your saliva; swallow it to make your *Qi* descend to your Cinnabar Field. Ingest your saliva that has been energized by the sun about nine times.

This habit will benefit sexual ability and digestion, as well as increasing spiritual tranquility.

Massaging the Cinnabar Field

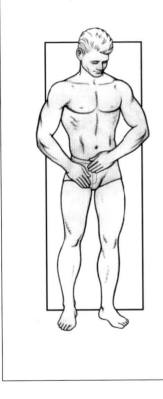

The Cinnabar Field, or dantian, is the center of gravity and core of energy of the body. It is found between the pubis and the belly button (point 8).

As with the previous exercise, massaging the Cinnabar Field increases sexual potency. This is an exercise that men must practice.

Using the palms of your hands, apply pressure slowly, deeply, and in an upward motion to the inside of your left thigh, near the groin (point 13). Next, move on to the right thigh. Finish by applying downward pressure toward the lower dantian or the perineum. Apply pressure about thirty-six times in each spot.

This is a well-rounded exercise because aside from increasing sexual energy, it also prevents impotence and, since it stimulates the prostate, increases fertility.

BOLSTERING THE SPERM

By using these exercises, you will thicken your sperm, increase sexual prowess, and improve fertility. The ideal time to do these exercises is during the night, specifically between 11 pm and 10 am.

1. While standing up and wearing just enough clothing to stay warm, rub your hands together until they are warm.

2. Transfer the heat from your hands to your testicles and your Cinnabar Field by holding your scrotum with one hand and pressing down on your belly button with the other.

3. While applying pressure, you must focus your mind on your suprarenal glands, which are just above the kidneys. Remain concentrated in this position for about ten minutes. By focusing the mind on a specific part of the body, energy is accumulated inside and transformed into substance (in this case, semen).
If you do this every day, you will begin to experience the benefits after about three months.

THE RED DRAGON

These exercises for men help to prolong erection and increase the amount of male hormones.

1. Kneel down without sitting on your feet, and keep your back straight. Gently squeeze your scrotum with your left hand. Breathe deeply, allowing the air to flow toward your lower dantian.

2. Breathe in and hold the air. Without exhaling, use the middle finger of your right hand to press down on the *huiyin* point, located in the middle of the perineum (see page 62). Try to grit your teeth and apply pressure with your tongue to the base of your upper row of teeth. This helps with concentration.

3. At the same time as you are pressing your *huiyin* point, you should vigorously clench your anus and lean your chest slightly forward without bending your back and contracting your abdomen. Lower yourself until your buttocks are about two inches away from your feet, and hold this position while clenching your anus and holding your breath for about five seconds.

4. Relax all your muscles while you slowly exhale and rest your buttocks on your feet.

Repeat this exercise five times a day. The best time to do this is in the morning after you wake up or at night before going to sleep. When you master this technique, you will be able to move your penis at will because the muscles of the anus and penis are connected. Clenching one will cause both to move. It will take three months of consistent practice to start experiencing the benefits of this exercise. Exercises that allow for a longer erection time and an increase in sexual vigor require persistence and determination. Once you master this technique, maintaining your sexual potency will become much easier.

When you wake up in the morning with an erection, hold your penis in your hand and breathe deeply. As you breathe in, clench your anus and hold your penis firmly. You will feel it expand. Breathe out, let go of your penis, and relax your anal muscles. Repeat this exercise thirty-six times.

Exercises for women

ABSORBING THE ENERGY OF THE MOON

The best lunar phase for absorbing the moon's *Qi* is the full moon. Regardless of the moon's phase, it is best to absorb its *Qi* just after it has risen by standing in front of it while devoid of clothing.

Once you are facing the moon, breathe deeply. You will notice saliva gathering in your mouth. Swallow it now that it is impregnated with lunar energy. Remain facing the moon until you have swallowed about thirty times.

The energy of the moon, in the form of saliva, or *Jing* (substance), will become sexual energy (*Qi*) in the Cinnabar Field. Remember that the Three Treasures (*Qi, Jing,* and *Shen*) are all able to transform into one another. This way, you will experience an increase in your sexual energy and your vitality in general, as well as your spiritual tranquility.

The sexually stimulating *huiyin* point

The *huiyin* point is located in the center of the perineum, the region between the anus and the genitals.

This point is connected to the clitoris in such a way that by stimulating it, the clitoris also becomes aroused. Chinese shiatsu (acupressure) techniques, when applied to the *huiyin* point, create arousal before the act of sex begins. More importantly though, when done regularly, they increase sexual energy as well as the intensity of pleasure. The technique for women who wish to increase their sexual vigor and take pleasure in their relationships is as follows. Press deeply upon the *huiyin* point with your middle finger in an upward motion and forward toward the clitoris until you feel pain. Relax the pressure without losing contact between your finger and the point. Repeat the cycle every day for about ten minutes.

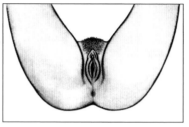

URINATING ON TIP TOES

This exercise, in the case of women, increases the strength of the love muscle, which also controls micturition and sex. When urinating, it expands outward and downward and contracts inward and upward when holding in urine. You may also find it by observing the anus. When you strain the love muscle outward and downward, you will notice your anus widening. On the other hand, when you clench it upward and inward the anal opening will close.

This exercise will develop both expansion and contraction. The technique consists of forcing urination by applying pressure to the lower abdomen, which causes the flow of urine to increase. Using Western toilets hinders this exercise, so it will be necessary to adapt to the circumstances.

While sitting on the toilet, place your feet on your fingers and lean forward while gritting your teeth and pressing your lower abdomen down and back, causing urine to be expelled with force.

There is also another technique to complement this one: while you are urinating, interrupt your stream suddenly by forcefully clenching the anus. This contraction will reach all the way to the clitoris. You will have mastered this technique when not a single drop of urine escapes after clenching.

It is recommended to alternate interrupting the flow of urine and forcing it once or twice every time you relieve yourself.

These exercises, when combined with the following technique, considerably strengthen the muscles of the vagina, the anus, and the clitoris (all three of which together are called the "love muscle") and noticeably increase the sexual potency of those who do them.

EXERCISES FOR THE VAGINA

These exercises develop the love muscle using contractions directed inward and upward.

The basic exercise consists of clenching the anus and vagina with force, so that the contraction reaches the clitoris, while breathing in through the nose and keeping the tongue pressed against the base of the upper row of teeth. Follow up by exhaling through the mouth and relaxing all your muscles. You can do this exercise in any place or position. The more you practice, the better. You may also complement the exercise by adding elements that work out the abdomen and hips.

1. Lie down on the ground face up with your arms on either side of your body and your palms resting on the floor. Slightly lift your hips without bending your knees while breathing in through your nose and clenching your anus and vagina. Exhale through the mouth while relaxing your muscles and lowering your hips. Repeat this exercise fifteen times.

2. Lie down face up with knees bent and the bottoms of your feet on the ground. Lift your hips while breathing in and contracting your love muscle. Relax your muscles while you exhale and bring your hips back down. Repeat this exercise fifteen times.

3. Remain on the ground, stretch your legs, cross them, and place your feet on a wall at ground height without lifting your legs. In this position, lift your hips, pelvis, and head at the same time while inhaling and contracting your anal and vaginal muscles. Lower your head and hips, relax your muscles, and breathe. Repeat this sequence fifteen times.

For women who have just given birth, there are specific exercises that help tone the vaginal muscles. Western doctors have adapted Chinese vaginal exercises for this purpose. The woman must place an appropriately sized heavy object in her vagina and hold it using the muscles located there so that it cannot fall. Do not hesitate to call your gynecologist if you wish to obtain the weights and start exercising.

Exercises of the White Tigresses

ABSORBING THE BREATH OF THE DRAGON

This is one of the main techniques of transformation. The Tigresses have two ways of doing it:

1. Tightly closing the legs when the man is about to achieve orgasm to prevent any waste of *Qi*.

2. Placing the head of the penis in her mouth and inhaling nine times. With each exhale, she must clench her anus. Upon doing this, the Tigress must visualize the energy in the form of green vapor emanating from the penis and allow it to flow into her head.

The Tigresses are prudent. They only practice certain exercises with their Jade Dragon, and they will not engage in certain risky practices with Green Dragons, which includes receiving semen in dangerous areas. Also, if they do not trust the Dragon for whatever reason, they will immediately leave the encounter.

In cases where the Green Dragon is trustworthy (these days, the only way to be sure is by medically testing for STDs), the Tigress will move forward with the absorption. She will move her tongue in circles around the head of the man's penis while it is still in her mouth. At this point, she generates a large amount of saliva and extracts the tears of the Dragon, the fluid that is secreted by men before ejaculating. The Tigress mixes the two fluids in her mouth as she sucks on the Dragon's penis and allows them to flow over the length of her tongue eighteen times. Then, she swallows the fluid hard in such a way that she can feel it reaching her abdomen. If the Tigress feels a slight vibration in the lower part of her abdomen, it means the process is going very well and she will enjoy multiple benefits.

Tigresses tend to avail themselves of manual techniques in order to bring the Dragon to orgasm. Using the hands to stimulate is a technique similar to oral sex and is considered an effective secondary form of stimulation.

The Tigress caresses the base of the penis with one hand while stimulating it with the other. She may also bring her head close in order to open her mouth, extend her tongue, and gently brush it. She may also rotate her hand around the head of the penis, wrap her hair around it, and masturbate him using both hands.

Absorbing the breath of the Dragon leads Tigresses to another technique of transformation: illumination. Tigresses must use their energy to see small lights in their minds that move slowly and in harmony. After an encounter with a Dragon, the Tigress will sit and meditate in order to reach this state.

TOUCHING THE SCALES OF THE DRAGON

This is a very effective masturbatory technique. The man must remain seated with legs apart while the woman kneels between them. The woman will carefully insert the ring finger of her left hand into the man's anus to stimulate the *huiyin* area (an energy core). She will then stroke the base of the penis with the index finger and thumb of the same hand.

With her right hand spread with oil, the Tigress will stimulate the head of the penis slowly and firmly using circular motions. The rhythm will be slow, since the purpose is for the man to reach orgasm using his mind more than the physical actions of his Tigress. This method gives the man a very intense and drawn-out orgasm.

The act of sex

The act of sex does not consist solely of penetration. It is an activity that must be done completely, including foreplay, which is as pleasurable as it is necessary. Omitting foreplay and rushing toward orgasm is like reading the last page of a book before the first. In sex, there is not a goal or a need to obtain something. It should be enjoyed in full in a way that enriches the body and mind.

Rushing toward it will only result in failing to achieve pleasure. Every step previous to penetration and orgasm is full of enjoyment. Strokes, kisses, touches, small scratches, licks, goose bumps... Think of when you were still a virgin, and remember the pleasure of a simple touch without penetration.

Reducing all the steps of the journey into a single one is to cheapen the sexual act and rob it of enjoyment. It is like simply driving to a destination instead of walking a path and experiencing every beautiful and tranquil moment. Sure, you may reach your destination sooner in the first case, but ultimately, was that really your goal?

In order to experience sex fully and completely, Taoists determined that there were certain indicators that had to be present before initiating it. The absence of said signs meant that penetration should be postponed.

One must keep in mind that rushing not only reduces pleasure but, in many cases, also prevents the woman from reaching orgasm, an unfortunate outcome for the couple. Additionally, the man's health is impacted due to the loss of energy during ejaculation that can only be recovered by absorbing fluids that the woman emits during sex and her own orgasm.

For the woman to reach orgasm, it is essential that penetration happen at the height of her arousal and never sooner. It is better to begin penetration when the woman is at the cusp of reaching orgasm than to start too soon and then try later, with great effort, to delay ejaculation.

The woman's Five Signs

The *Tao* lends great importance to the woman's pleasure. Because of this, a great deal of effort was invested in studying women's sexual responses during the act of sex so that men could know if their partners were enjoying themselves.

Women may present five signs that they are feeling pleasure. That is not to say that all five signs are always present or in the same order, but they can be used as a guide for men to interpret what their partners' bodies are telling them.

- **First Desire or Intent.** Breathing and pulse are accelerated. The man may approach the woman.
- **Second Desire or Consciousness.** The nostrils are tense, and the mouth is half open. The man must stroke the woman's body and stimulate the genitals.
- **Third Desire.** There is an abundance of vaginal fluids, arousal is very evident, and the woman is holding on tightly to the man's body. Penetration may begin.
- **Fourth Desire or Concentration.** Female orgasm. Breathing becomes jarred, and the woman is sweating profusely.
- **Fifth Desire.** A stronger than normal orgasm. The woman's body becomes rigid and exerts pressure against the man while the eyes are closed.

Next, we will look at some useful techniques for letting the energy of love flow, for men to be in adequate physical shape for initiating sex (or the Four Successes), and understanding the signs that will guide them during the act (the Five Desires, the ten Indicators, and the Five Signs).

Massage. With massage, couples are able to open their gates or energy cores and stimulate the circulation of energy through the meridians. This way, they also prepare their bodies for the great exchange of energy that is produced during sex.

Massage eliminates each lover's individuality and allows both participants to become so close that they become as one body. This union is fundamentally important for the valuable exchange of energy and substances between the pair.

Important: To those who have read this far, we recommend developing the massage techniques presented on page 107 and the pages that follow.

Pressure on the *Triple Yin* intersection point

This massage is worth learning because of the highly arousing effect it has on women. Locate the *Triple Yin* (*San Yin Jiao*) intersection point, found behind the

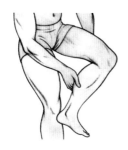 calf bone about three inches away from the inner ankle bone. Hold the calf with one hand, with your thumb resting on the point, and press down until there is pain. Relax the pressure without losing contact between your finger and the point. Repeat these steps several times. You can apply this pressure yourself or with the help of your partner.

Foot massage

This is a very stimulating massage for men because it positively affects the liver, which is the organ that sends the additional blood necessary for erection. Hold the first foot in both hands, and rub the entire bottom, as well as the toes. Repeat this same process with the other foot. This massage must be deep and vigorous.

Requirements for beginning coitus

The Mysterious Girl, sexual adviser to the Yellow Emperor, one of the founders of the Chinese civilization who ruled until the year 2700 B.C., is clearly quoted in this passage gathered by Lao Tse:

MYSTERIOUS GIRL: A man who desires copulation must first achieve the Four Successes: extension, thickening, hardening, and heat.

YELLOW EMPEROR: What do these achievements mean?

MYSTERIOUS GIRL: If the stem does not reach the required length, then the man's energy is too exhausted for the act. If he is long enough but not thick enough, this means that his muscular energy is insufficient for the task. If he achieves thickness but not hardness, then his joints and tendons are too weak for the act. If the member hardens but does not become warm, he does not have enough spirit for the act. In order to be fully prepared for sex, the muscles and bones must first be in harmony with the spirit and energy. One must also exercise restraint, according to the basic principle of *Tao*, and not waste semen for any reason.

In this fragment, the Mysterious Girl not only shows what the man requires in order to initiate sex, but she also explains that sexual health is only present in bodies that benefit from good health in general (physical and mental). The passage also emphasizes the intimate relation among the Three Treasures and the importance of taking equal care of all of them.

The man adapts to the rhythm of the woman

The man must adapt to the woman's requirements for initiating sex. Western thinking tends to promote the idea that it is the man who sets the rhythm during coitus. Contrary to this, Taoism shows that fulfilling sex is directed by the desires of the woman.

She sets the pace through subtle suggestions that the man must recognize. In addition to the Five Wishes, the man may interpret his partner's sexual demands through the Ten Indicators and the Five Signs.

The Ten Indicators are conscious reactions by which the woman directs the man's actions during sex, when verbal communication is difficult. If the man follows these directions, he will be able to avail himself of the fluids that will become sexual energy in his own body. In addition to the increase in energy, there will be an increase in concentration and understanding between the couple.

The Ten Indicators

- **First Indicator.** The woman clings to the man with arms and legs to make contact between the genitals possible.
- **Second Indicator.** The woman shyly caresses the man's genitals. He, in turn, should use his fingers to stroke her clitoris and vaginal opening.
- **Third Indicator.** The woman arches her spine while throwing her head back, opening her mouth, and spreading her legs wide. Begin penetration.
- **Fourth Indicator.** Her whole body trembles, which is a sign that she is feeling pleasure.
- **Fifth Indicator.** The woman wraps her legs around the man, indicating that he should move with greater vigor.
- **Sixth Indicator.** The woman presses herself harder against the man to make penetration deeper. At this time she is approaching orgasm, and the man must not lose his rhythm.
- **Seventh Indicator.** She moves her hips from side to side. The man must alternate his penetrations, directing them to the left and to the right.
- **Eighth Indicator.** The woman strains her whole body and presses herself against the man. He must continue moving constantly and vigorously because her orgasm is beginning.
- **Ninth Indicator.** Female orgasm. The woman's entire body is tense.
- **Tenth Indicator.** The Lunar Flower, the essence emitted by the woman during orgasm, flows out. The man may withdraw his penis and approach with his tongue to swallow this valuable fluid.

Lastly, the Five Signs indicate at what stage of pleasure the woman finds herself during copulation. These signs are all physical and easily identified. They are greatly useful to men because they make it possible for them to match their rhythm to the woman's, which makes it easier to reach simultaneous orgasm.

The Five Signs

- **First Sign.** The woman's face reddens. She is feeling sexual desire, which indicates that the man may begin caressing the Mound of Venus with his own member.
- **Second Sign.** Her nipples harden, and small beads of sweat appear around her nose. She is aroused enough to be penetrated.
- **Third Sign.** Her throat and lips are dry, which makes it hard to swallow. She is approaching orgasm, and the man must move with greater force.
- **Fourth Sign.** The Jade Portal (vaginal opening) moistens. She is entering orgasm. The man must penetrate deeply and move from side to side.
- **Fifth Sign.** A viscous liquid runs down the thighs; the orgasm has ended, and the man may withdraw.

Controlling ejaculation

According to Taoism, each male ejaculation brings with it a considerable loss of primordial energy, which decreases steadily until it disappears at the time of death.

The man must avoid accelerating this process by reserving his semen and replenishing his stores of energy by absorbing the libations of the Three Peaks, which are essences secreted by the woman during sex.

Taoists know of techniques for retaining semen during orgasm and reabsorbing it so that it may become *Qi* and *Shen*. Knowing how the flow of energy within the organism works helps to extend genital orgasms throughout the whole body and allows the use of vital or sexual energy for creative and curative purposes.

When faced with the greatest tenet of Taoism that says the path of nature is the right path, one may ask if containing semen is natural or not. A man produces an amount of semen or vital fluid each day, but if he does not need to replenish his sperm, according to the *Tao*, this energy may be used to increase spiritual growth and fortify the mind and body.

In order to learn Taoist techniques and experience multiple orgasms without ejaculating, the man must learn to control his sexual energy, which is concentrated in most cases within the genitals, and make it flow throughout his whole body. Following this, the Western man must determine what his sexual frequencies are according to the dictates of his own organism. He must be capable of distinguishing between sincere and artificial sexual desires because no instruction manual may show him his own optimal sexual frequency.

To give an example of the uniqueness of each case, let's read what the Simple Girl said to the Yellow Emperor:

> There are strong men, as there are weak men. Each one must live with his own vitality, as it is detrimental to try to force pleasure.
>
> A young healthy man of twenty years may ejaculate twice a day, but if he is weak, he should do it no more than once daily.
>
> At thirty years he may ejaculate once a day, or every other day if his energy is weak.
>
> At forty years old, he will be able to ejaculate once every three days, or once every four if he is sickly.
>
> A strong man of fifty years may issue his semen once every five days, or once every ten if he is weak.
>
> A sixty-year-old man may ejaculate once every ten days if he is healthy, and once every twenty if he is not.
>
> At seventy years of age, if he conserves his strength, a man may ejaculate once a month. Otherwise, he must conserve his semen permanently from then on.

If a man learns to achieve orgasm without the need to ejaculate, he will never tire; the feeling he would normally have after sex (exhaustion, lethargy, and weakness) will disappear and become energy that may bolster health and pleasure.

Jolan Chang, in *The Tao of Love and Sex*, said of pleasure without ejaculation:

> I am frequently asked what pleasure can be had if one only ejaculates once for every hundred orgasms. I generally respond thusly: I would not exchange the intense pleasure that I feel with yours. The twelve years during which I was obsessed with obtaining pleasure at the time of ejaculation are, for me, long wasted years. If my interlocutor is a man, he cannot doubt my sincerity, for he sees me placid, happy, in good health, and always in the mood to make love. . . . Now I can say that sex without ejaculation also represents the elimination of tension, but without an explosion. It is a pleasure produced through appeasement, not violence. It is a voluptuous, sensual, and prolonged fusion that transcends entirely beyond oneself. It is a feeling of communion with everything, not separation; of participation and union, rather than a solitary and individual spasm that excludes the partner. There are no words to describe it.

Techniques to control ejaculation

CLOSED METHOD

This is the most ancient method for learning to control ejaculation, which was written by the Taoist Wu Hsien. It requires no great ability nor effort.

Upon penetrating a woman, the man must make one deep movement and three superficial movements while closing his eyes and mouth and breathing deeply through his nose without panting. When he is on the verge of losing control, he should withdraw his penis by up to an inch and remain still. Then, he will breathe deeply and contract the lower part of his stomach as if he were holding in his urine. He should concentrate on how he must not let his precious semen escape. When he regains control, he will be ready to continue without having lost firmness or semen. With practice, he will be able to better control his ejaculation.

PRESSURE METHOD

This technique can be used in any position, and the man applies it to himself. Using the index and middle fingers of his left hand, the man presses on the point located between the scrotum and the anus for three or four seconds each time he inhales.

The advantage of this method is that the man does not need to stop, which allows the woman to continue receiving pleasure.

Penetration techniques

When the Third Desire, the Third Indicator, and the Second Sign become evident in the woman and the Four Successes in the man, penetration may commence.

To begin, the man must push gently until he has comfortably entered his partner. He will continue thrusting superficially, face to face with his partner, while brushing the clitoris with the base of his penis and keeping friction upon the gland to a minimum.

This technique gives pleasure to the woman while keeping the man calm.

The penetrative techniques to follow will depend on the signals given by the woman. Lin Tung-Hsuan, a doctor from the Tang dynasty, explains some of these techniques:

Use the base of the Jade Stem (penis) as if it were a saw, exerting upward and downward pressure upon the mound above the Jade Portal (vaginal opening). Try to reach the Precious Pearl (clitoris) that resides inside the oyster.

Sink the Jade Stem deep within the Jade Portal and then slowly withdraw it, letting it drag the Golden Hollow (upper vulva) with it, as if it were trying to absorb the female Yin essence.

Use the Jade Stem as a mortar, pressing vigorously down on the Jade Terrace (clitoris) and receiving medicinal essences.

Penetrate until reaching the Celestial Palace (upper vagina) and, without exiting it, make short and slow pushes, as if planting seeds in a field.

Rub the Jade Stem against the Jade Portal with the strength of two colliding avalanches. Penetrate towards the left and right, as if fighting with a sword against a great band of warriors.

Move the Jade Stem up and down, like a wild horse crossing a stream.

Alternate between deep and shallow penetrations, all of them slow, while keeping the rhythm of a stone tossed into the sea.

Slowly insert the Jade Stem into the Jade Portal, mimicking the slithering movement of a snake entering the burrow of its prey.

Now penetrate quickly, like a mouse scurrying to safety upon sensing danger.

Lift the head of the Stem high and plunge it downwards, in a movement similar to the prow of a ship battered by a storm.

We can also differentiate between two techniques depending on the depth of penetration.

- **Superficial push.** Only half of the penis enters, which produces friction between the gland of the penis and the G-spot inside the vagina (the woman may locate this spot if she introduces her index finger into her vagina up to the first phalange and presses against her anterior wall). If the man is penetrating from behind, he must push downward and the woman should lean her pelvis back. If they are face to face, the man will push upward and the woman will lean her pelvis forward.

- **Deep push.** The penis is inserted as deep as possible so that there is friction between the base of the penis and the clitoris. If the couple is facing each other, the man exerts upward pressure with his penis and the woman leans her pelvis back. If facing away from each other, the man will press the base of his penis against the woman's perineum (opposite her clitoris, between the vagina and anus) and the woman will push downward while leaning the pelvis forward and causing her back to arch.

Penetrative technique of the White Tigress. White Tigresses do not base their sexual encounters around penetration nor do they usually allow men to enter them because it is not the most effective way of obtaining energy. Additionally, penetration is not beneficial to the vagina, which, according to their beliefs, should be relaxed. When tigresses allow penetration, normally with their Jade Dragon, they only take in the head of the penis.

It is believed that the following technique rejuvenates the Dragon, as well as the Tigress.

TAKING THE PEACH OF IMMORTALITY

The peach is associated with the virginal vagina in Chinese culture. During this section, we take into account the same considerations expressed in "Freezing the Jade Dragon" (page 49). The woman lies down on the bed with her head on a pillow and another pillow under her bottom while the Jade Dragon sits between her legs. There should be silence, tranquility, and a bit of incense.

The Jade Dragon inserts his finger up to the first knuckle into the woman's vagina. She places her hands, forming cups over her breasts and moves her hips while trying to force his finger deeper inside her. He does not allow it to happen.

When the Tigress is wet, the man climbs on top and inserts the head of his penis into her vagina. She gyrates her hips while trying to force him deeper inside, but he maintains the distance and prevents deeper penetration.

With her hands still on her breasts, she offers her nipples to the Jade Dragon, and he stimulates them with circular motions of his tongue and light sucking.

When she is nearing orgasm, she will signal the Jade Dragon. They will switch positions, and he will be on the bottom with her on top. She will place her vagina over his mouth, swallow as much of his penis as she can, and remain this way. He will suck on her vagina and swallow all of her juices as they flow from her. When she reaches orgasm, she will let go of his penis and make a "haa" sound while at the same time pressing her vagina against his mouth so he may continue receiving her libations. Then, he will place his tongue against his teeth and mix her fluids with his saliva thirty-six times. He will swallow this mixture in three equal portions.

If the Jade Dragon reaches orgasm, the Tigress will direct his essence onto her face and leave it there until the exercise is over. If she cannot reach orgasm during this session, they will try again during another. When they separate, they will sit in meditation and try to reach illumination.

Sex positions

There are a number of sex positions, and they are all derived from three basic figures that allow different variations.

- **Man behind the woman.** This position allows for deeper penetration and greater friction between the penis and the walls of the vagina. Pressure exerts on the G-spot, which is located on the front wall of the vagina about the distance of one phalange from the middle finger when starting at the vaginal opening. Stimulating this spot creates intense pleasure for the woman. This position may seem basic, but it is the most pleasurable. However, it is not recommended for men who suffer from premature ejaculation.

- **Woman on top of man.** The woman sits on top of the man while introducing his penis into her vagina. This position stimulates the clitoris and allows the woman to control the depth of penetration. It is recommended for men who ejaculate prematurely and for women who are afraid of feeling pain during penetration or want to follow their own rhythm.

- **Face to face.** This posture allows the couple to add additional stroking and kissing to the act, but given that it prevents deep penetration and hinders the woman's movement, it is reserved for the beginning of the session and switched shortly after starting. Men who ejaculate prematurely should not risk losing control during such an unsatisfying position for the woman.

In every posture, the woman must move her pelvis backward and forward to find the angle of penetration that feels the most pleasurable. One variation that feels very good for the woman is, while she is lying on her back, for the man to raise his body up higher than normal and place his elbows on the surface the woman is lying on over her shoulders. While the man is higher up than the woman, his penis exerts an enjoyable amount of pressure on her clitoris.

Out of the many positions there are, we will emphasize the ones that the Simple Girl explained to the Yellow Emperor, which are called the Nine Methods and are considered to be generally curative for the man as much as for the woman.

- **The spinning dragon.** The woman lies face down with her legs spread. The man, on his knees and elbows, gets down on top of her. The penis should softly caress the clitoris, which incites greater arousal in his partner, and then penetrate the vagina while thrusting deeply one time for every eight shallow thrusts. Next, the man will gyrate his hips, causing friction between the base of his penis and the upper part of the vaginal opening.

- **The stalking tiger.** The woman is on her hands and knees with the man behind her, also on his knees, holding her by the hips. The rhythm of penetration will vary according to the woman's signals.

- **The jumping monkey.** The woman lies face up with her legs spread, and the man crouches toward her and grabs her hips. She raises her legs and places them on his shoulders. If the woman lies down on the edge of a table, the man will be able to approach her while standing and the position will be somewhat more comfortable.

- **The mating cicadas.** The woman starts off in a crawling position, and the man approaches from behind on his knees. Once the couple has comfortably achieved penetration, the woman will stretch her legs out while the man lies down on top of her while holding his weight with his hands to avoid restricting her breathing. In this comfortable position, the man will make six deep thrusts and one shallow one or nine deep thrusts and one shallow one.

■ **The turtle that mounts.** The woman lies face up, bends her knees, and brings them toward her breasts. The man approaches on his knees and leans on the back of her thighs, which are in the air in such a way that the woman may rest her calves on his arms. The man should alternate between shallow and deep thrusts and increase the speed and force of penetration during the woman's orgasm.

■ **The flapping phoenix.** The woman lies face up with her legs separated and knees slightly bent while the man is on his hands and knees. He should combine a sequence of eight shallow thrusts followed by one deep one with a sequence of three shallow thrusts followed by one deep thrust.

■ **The rabbit that licks its hair.** The man lies face up and the woman mounts him while facing toward his feet and opening her legs and leaning slightly forward.

■ **The fish with overlapping scales.** The man lies face up with his legs stretched out and the woman on top. Penetration will start softly and then vary in depth and intensity according to the woman's desires. During penetration, the man will absorb libations from the woman's middle and upper peaks (breasts and tongue).

■ **The cranes with intertwining necks.** The man sits on a chair with his back straight and the woman mounts him, face to face, with her arms on his shoulders and her feet on the ground. The woman will control the thrusts by lifting herself while the man helps by holding her buttocks. It is more effective if the woman controls the action while the man holds the weight.

Curative positions

The act of sex is not just a source of pleasure and an exchange of energy. Sexuality may also be used for therapeutic purposes and is a valuable treatment for a number of ailments.

Curing sexual ailments through coitus

■ **Entering smoothly.** This technique treats male impotency and should be combined with a good diet, exercise, and a positive outlook free of anxiety and fear. With regards to the last requirement, meditation can be of great help, as it empties the mind and creates spiritual peace.

The man penetrates with a flaccid penis and moves it around inside the vagina until the right consistency is achieved. This position requires the collaboration of the female partner and for her to be considerably lubricated.

The man makes a circle with his thumb and index finger and holds the base of his penis to aid in penetration.

This technique is useful in cases of impotence where there is an erection but it does not last long enough.

■ **Cure for the Seven Evils.** The Simple Girl explains to the Yellow Emperor that those who abuse sex become ill due to an excessive loss of essence (semen). Illnesses born of this indiscretion are known as the Seven Evils: absence of desire, impotence, nocturnal emissions, anemia, lack of energy, mental weakness, and low hormone levels. The cure is the same for all the illnesses and consists of having sex several times a day for ten days with the same woman without ejaculating. The best time to use this cure is from midnight until dawn, and the best positions are those in which the man lies face up while the woman controls the pace as she sits on top. This allows for a greater retention of semen due to the effects of gravity at the time of ejaculation.

■ **Premature ejaculation.** The woman lies down on her side with her hips angled so they are pointing upward as much as possible. The man lies on top of her and performs two sequences of one shallow thrust followed by nine deep ones.

This position helps with impotence, premature ejaculation, and difficulties achieving orgasm.

By doing this, the man's amount of hormones will increase due to frequent sexual arousal, but he will not lose energy thanks to the lack of ejaculation.

Curing sexual ailments through coitus. Different parts of the vagina and penis are connected to the internal organs of the body, such as with the bottoms of the feet. For this reason, we can treat illnesses of the body through coitus by selecting the sexual position that best exerts pressure on the points related to the organs that need treatment.

The energy cores of the sex organs

Chinese tradition connects different areas of the penis and vagina with specific points on the body. The curing of ailments may be achieved by using positions that provide pressure to the correct areas.

PENIS

Gland. It is connected to the brain and ganglia.

Upper part of the penis next to the gland. It mirrors the lungs and heart.

Middle part. It is connected to the liver and spleen.

Base of the penis. It is linked to the kidneys.

VAGINA

Cervix. It correlates with the heart and lungs.

Upper part of the vagina (deeper zone). It corresponds to the spleen, pancreas, and stomach.

Middle part. It is linked to the liver.

Outer area. It is related to the kidneys.

Once we know which parts of the sex organs correspond with the inner parts of the body, we can choose the curative sexual position that best suits each couple. To achieve results, it helps to practice the chosen position at least once a day. The main curative positions are the following:

Positions for women

■ **Treating fatigue and weakness.** The woman lies down on her back, and the man lies on top of her with his weight on his elbows. The man penetrates her as deeply as he can while the woman moves her pelvis while alternating between clockwise and counterclockwise directions.

The woman decides when it is time to move on to something else either because she has reached orgasm or because she is in the mood for a different position. Reaching orgasm is not necessary for the effectiveness of these positions.

This position helps with lack of energy, excessive perspiration, weakness, palpitations, and blurred vision.

■ **Bodily cleansing.** The man lies on his back and the woman climbs on top while resting on her knees and facing his feet. Only the head of the penis needs to penetrate. The woman can then hold it in her hand to better control insertion. The woman should gyrate in both directions as much as she can.

This posture prevents the retention of fluids (very common in women), high fevers, kidney and bladder problems, and illnesses of the pituitary gland.

■ **Toning the internal organs.** The woman sits on top of a thick cushion and places her hands on her hips. The man kneels before her while supporting himself with one hand and holding one of the woman's calves with the other.

The woman wraps her other leg around the man's body. She needs to angle her pelvis upward in order to receive the full benefits of the position.

This posture bolsters Qi, kidneys, the liver, the spleen, and the heart of both participants, especially the woman.

- **Headaches and menstrual problems.** The man lies down on his back, and the woman lies down on his right so that she is leaning on her right knee while her left leg stretches across his body. With her right hand she leans next to his head, and with her left she controls the depth of penetration, which should be mid-depth.

  This position helps clear the meridians and is effective for headaches, poor circulation, and menstrual problems (pain, amenorrhea, excessive flow...).

- **Strengthening the nervous system.** The man lies down on his back while the woman sits on her knees face to face with him. She must alternate between deep and shallow penetration and rotate her hips so that the penis massages the vagina.

  This position cures ulcers and boosts the nervous system, liver, and vision.

Positions for men

- **Energizing the body.** The woman lies on her back with her head and shoulders on a large cushion. The man positions himself on top of her on his hands and knees. He should alternate between deep and shallow thrusts. The couple must perform a series of nine penetrations three times a day for twenty days.

- **Cleansing the blood and revitalizing circulation.** The man lies down face up and the woman climbs on top, face to face, spreading her legs and putting her weight on her knees while keeping her body straight. The man controls the pace, moving his pelvis up and down. Penetration should be deep. The couple should use this position for at least ten days.

  This will correct bad circulation, hypertension, anemia, and other ailments of the blood.

- **Strengthening the bones.** The woman lies down on the left side of her body with her left leg bent at the knee so that it is as close as possible to her back. The man lies down in front of her and looks for the best angle at which to penetrate. He should alternate between deep and shallow thrusts. The couple must perform five series of nine penetrations five times a day for five days. This position strengthens the bones by helping to heal breaks and fractures and helps to alleviate arthritis.

- **Revitalizing the internal organs.** The man and woman lie down face to face. The woman keeps her lower leg stretched out and bends her upper leg backward, while the man penetrates her using a series of nine shallow and deep thrusts. The position should be composed of four series of nine penetrations done at most four times a day for twenty days.

Relieving pain for both members

The man climbs on top of the woman, who is lying face up and wraps her arms and legs around the man. Penetration in this posture will be superficial. This position bolsters the joints and relieves pain in both halves of the couple. Additionally, it stimulates the liver, the biliary vesicles, and the woman's spleen.

How to reach multiple orgasms

Tao has no form or aroma;
It cannot be seen or heard,
And it cannot be used up.

Discovering that one may achieve multiple orgasms is a wonderful experience. Ejaculating is not synonymous with orgasm. Unlike the orgasm, which is a feeling of absolute pleasure, ejaculation is simply a reflex in the lower spine that leads to the emission of semen. Having orgasms without ejaculating creates deeper states of pleasure and avoids the waste caused by loss of semen, thereby increasing vitality and longevity. Discovering the erogenous zones of your partner is very important because, as you become more sensitive to your lover's body, so, too, will you discover your own. Becoming a multi orgasmic man or woman leads to deeper levels of pleasure and more frequent intimate encounters.

As a man learns to control his ejaculation, he will discover resources to help him disassociate it with pleasure and orgasm. The key is in the pleasure muscle.

Discovering the pleasure muscle

The pubococcygeus muscle, also known as the PC, is, in reality, a group of muscles that travel from the pubic bone to the posterior bone, or coccyx. Its purpose is to halt the flow of urine, and it is essential for becoming a multi orgasmic being.

His PC

It is the muscle that controls ejaculation by pushing the semen through the penis and out of the body. Most importantly, though, the entire male orgasm depends on having a strong PC. If a man exercises his pubococcygeus muscle, he may have multiple orgasms without the need for ejaculation.

There are techniques for strengthening the PC, and using them will allow you to increase your sexual pleasure.

Finding the muscle

To begin, you must locate the pubococcygeus muscle (PC). This may be simple for some men, but a great number are not familiar with this part of the body. Together, the individual muscles may seem like one great mass: buttocks, abdomen, thighs, and PC. It is very important to find the PC muscle and isolate it from the rest of the body.

1. First, place one or two fingers behind your testicles. Pretend you are urinating, and try to halt the flow from the bladder. The muscle you have just used is the PC. If you felt it tense up and your testicles moved a little, then you have located it.
2. It is very important for your stomach and thigh muscles to remain inert, so if you felt them move, try again. Also keep in mind that you do not need to be erect in order to perform this exercise, so relax and let your penis respond naturally.

Flexing the muscle

1. Now that you have found the muscle, the next step is to flex the muscle twenty times three times a day. Maintain the contraction for a second or two each time before letting go.

2. You do not need to hold your finger against the muscle during this exercise. By now, you should be able to feel the muscle moving internally, although you may need to use your fingers to begin. In the future, you will be able to do this with ease.

3. Try to keep your breathing normal; don't hold your breath. As with any other muscle exercise, maintaining adequate respiration is very important.

4. Repeat this sequence three times a day for three weeks.

The great pressure. When you have done the previous exercise for three weeks, you will be ready to apply the great pressure, also known as the potent pressure or the mortal compression. Slowly clench your PC as tightly as you can for five seconds. Next, maintain the tension for a further five seconds if you can, and then slowly release the pressure during the last five seconds. You should be able to feel your PC muscle working.

Doing this might be a little hard at the beginning. Maybe you are only able to do one or two fifteen-second clenches before tiring. It's okay; try increasing as you go along until you can repeat the exercise ten times with each one lasting between ten and fifteen seconds. It might take you a few days or weeks to reach this point. You must not overexert yourself; simply learn to enjoy the process and keep pushing forward. Don't forget to do the three series of twenty clenches mentioned previously.

Her PC

In the woman's case, the PC also goes from the pubic bone to the posterior bone, or coccyx, at the spine. It surrounds the urethra, anus, and vagina. It is the muscle that helps hold and exert pressure on the penis while it is in the vagina. In this case, having a strong pubococcygeus muscle may increase the woman's pleasure, as well as that of her partner, and make her orgasms more intense.

There are some techniques that strengthen the pubococcygeus muscle; use them to intensify your sexual desire, make childbirth less painful, and, best of all, intensify your orgasms and become multi orgasmic.

Locating the muscle

Most women know the PC as the muscle they use to hold in urine when they cannot use the restroom. Next time you have to urinate, locate the muscle by preventing micturition using the pelvic muscles. If the pubococcygeus muscle is strong, you will be able to halt the flow of urine and then resume afterward. If urine begins dripping out while you are clenching, your PC is not strong enough.

It is very important for the stomach and thigh muscles to remain at ease. If you feel them tensing, you must begin again.

It is likely that at the start you may feel pinpricks when trying to halt urination. This is normal, and as you practice the exercise, the sensation will disappear.

Voluntary contractions. Once you have located the muscle, do the following exercise:

1. Breathe in, and focus your attention on your vagina. As you exhale, squeeze your PC muscle, as well as the muscles near your mouth and eyes.

2. Breathe in again, and relax your muscles. Remember that the most important thing is to clench and relax your pubococcygeus muscle as many times as possible.

3. Repeat the sequence a minimum of ten times and at most thirty-six times three times a day for three weeks. You may do this at any time.

Small clenches. If you have done the previous exercise for at least three weeks, you will be ready for the next step. You must clench your PC muscle, but this time you will use your fingers, those of your partner, or his penis. Contract your PC muscle while exerting

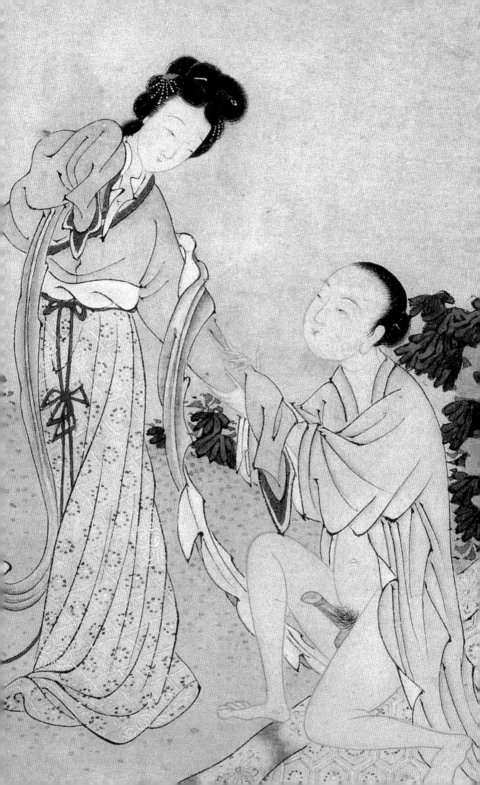

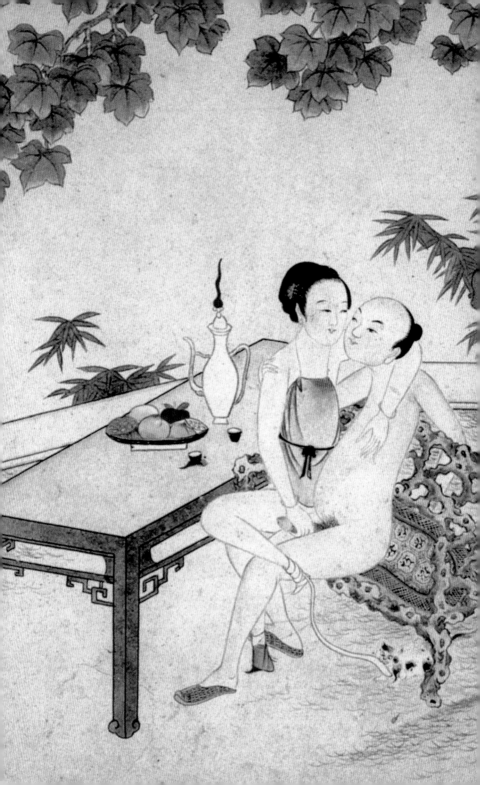

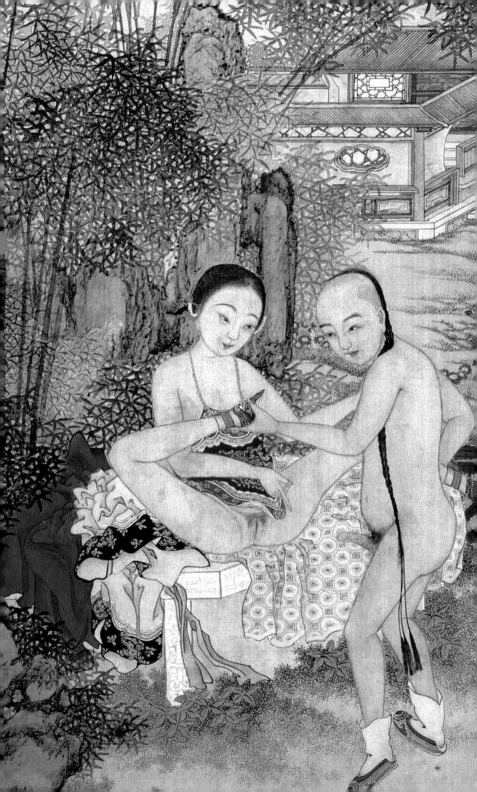

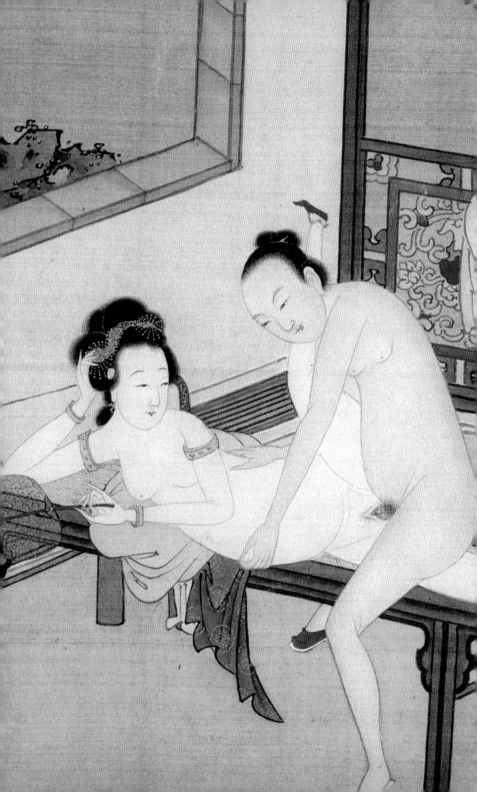

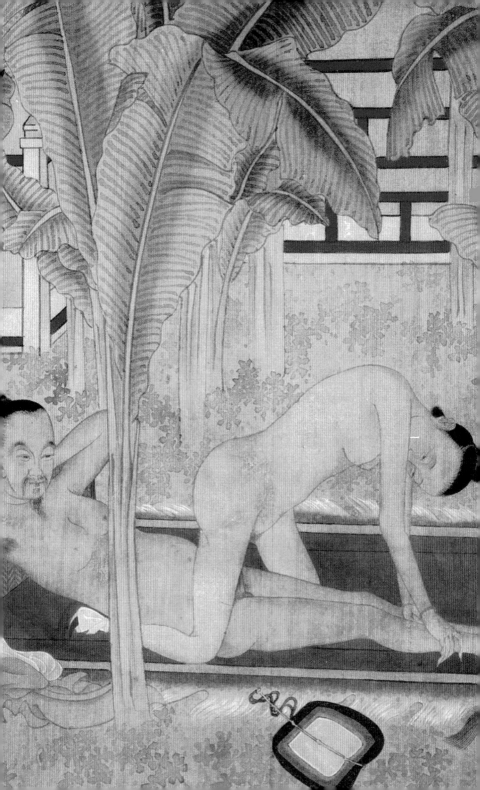

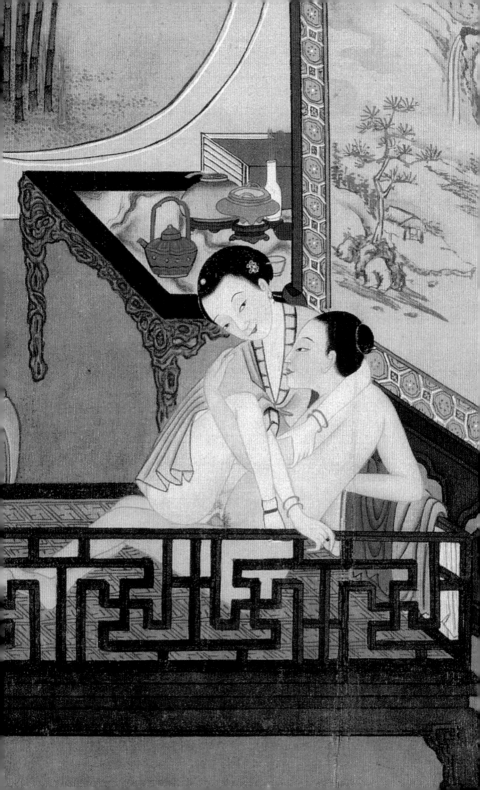

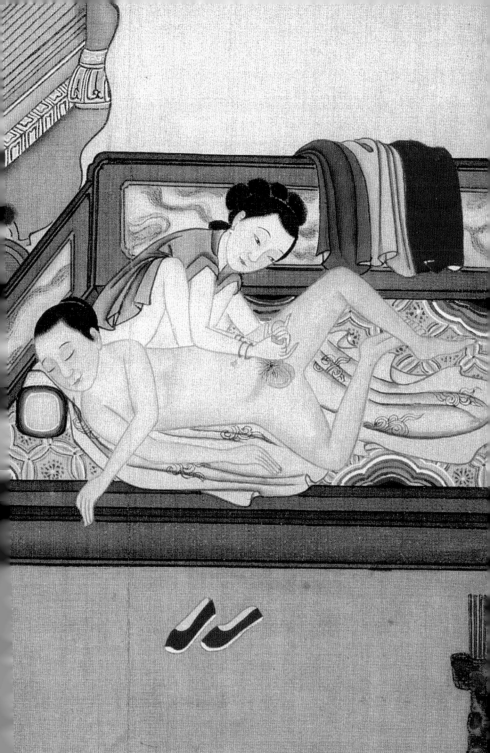

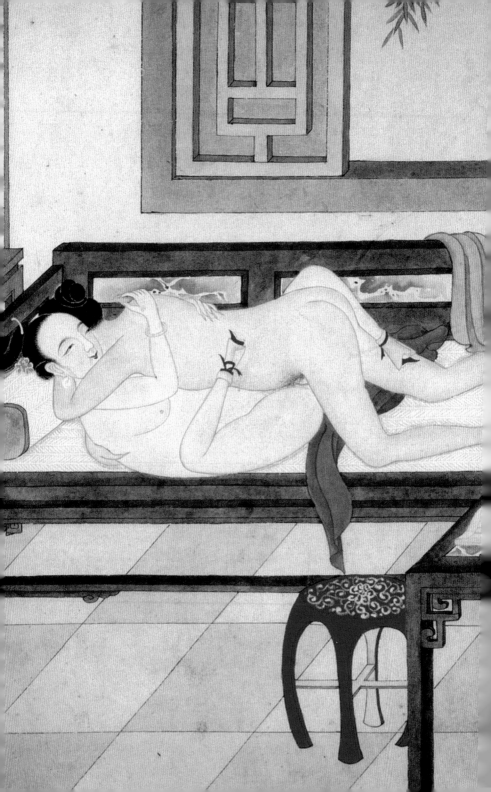

pressure on your fingers or those of your partner. You will clearly be able to feel if you are using the correct amount of force. The same thing happens if you squeeze the penis; your partner will be able to tell you if the pressure is strong. This sensation can be very pleasurable for both parties.

Becoming a multi-orgasmic man

The following exercise, to be practiced with your partner, teaches how to control ejaculation and start down the road toward becoming a multi orgasmic man.

1. During coitus, the woman may help the man become multi-orgasmic. First, she must stop moving when she feels that the man is approaching ejaculation and the height of arousal.

2. The man must change the rate of his breathing by making it either faster or slower. Slow breathing helps control sexual energy, and fast breathing allows the energy concentrated in the sexual organs to disperse.

3. It is important to circulate the energy. The woman must stroke the man's backbone with her hand from the coccyx up to the head. This makes the energy concentrated in the penis flow throughout the whole body.

4. The man can halt the emission of semen by pressing his perineum, located between the anus and testicles, at the same time as he clenches his PC muscle. It is possible for him to lose his erection using this method, but he may get it back quickly.

5. The woman may help delay male ejaculation using the following technique: Form a circle with your fingers and place them around the testicles. Then, pull on the testicles gently but firmly.

Becoming a multi-orgasmic woman

Female orgasms may be clitoral, vaginal, or both. One way of reaching orgasm more easily is by stimulating the clitoris during coitus. The clitoris is located under the Mound of Venus, where the inner lips join together. It is made of erectile tissue, like the penis, and fills with blood and increases in size when aroused.

It is very important that the man stimulate his partner's clitoris, as it is an easy way to bring her to orgasm. He must allow the woman to guide him by showing him where the clitoris is and what amount of pressure she enjoys. Some prefer to be stimulated with greater pressure while others enjoy soft and constant movements.

The G-spot is also a major area of arousal for women. To locate it, introduce your index or middle finger one or two inches and rub the anterior wall of the vagina. The spot is difficult to find, but it may be easier to locate after orgasm, when it increases in size.

It is best to stimulate the G-spot when the woman is approaching orgasm. It has been observed that waiting until then is more enjoyable than doing it at the beginning of sex.

Stimulating the G-spot is easier when the woman is lying face down and the man penetrates her from behind. In this posture, the penis grazes the G-spot, which explains why so many women prefer this sexual position.

The following exercises empower the multi-orgasmic being that exists inside each woman.

Pressing an egg

1. For this exercise, you need an egg-shaped object about two inches in diameter and two and a half inches long. It should be made of a non-porous and smooth material, such as quartz.

2. Before starting, make sure the egg is clean to prevent any sort of vaginal infection. To avoid the egg getting stuck inside the

vagina, you can make a hole in it and attach a string like on tampons.

3. In a comfortable position either sitting or standing, introduce the previously lubricated egg in the vagina, breathe in, and clench the PC muscle.

4. Exhale, loosen the PC muscle, and push the egg toward the vagina's exit without taking it completely out.

5. Repeat the exercise for at least five minutes and at most ten. When you are done, exhale forcefully and remove the egg.

Learning to feel oneself

1. The first thing you should do is learn where all your genital organs are located. Afterward, softly and in harmony with the universe around you, touch your clitoris, stroke the lips of your vagina, and begin experiencing the pleasure they bring your body.

2. Breathe slowly and become conscious of your respiration. When you exhale, clench your vagina.

3. As you do this exercise, think of your body as a great container of light and energy that opens up to the world like a flower blooming in the spring. Let the sensation of excitement you feel when you touch yourself flow through your body, and think about that energy rising from the base of your spine to your head.

4. If you have difficulties feeling the energy ascending from your coccyx to your brain, clench your anus and vagina until you feel the energy rising and spreading to your whole body, therefore creating a sensation of well-being.

Sensitive concentration

The sensitive concentration techniques are sexual contact exercises for men and women who wish to learn how to control and appreciate physical contact. They create a level of concentration that leads to an extraordinary amount of control over the different stages of arousal, orgasm, and ejaculation.

Becoming sensitive to the process of arousal is a very important step toward becoming multi orgasmic. Sensitive concentration focuses your mind and lets you enjoy every individual erotic aspect of your arousal and your partner's.

Preparing for the exercises

Do the following exercises in a quiet room where you will not be distracted. You will need a bed and a chair for doing the exercises alone if that is your preference. You must also have a little massage oil at hand or a different cream or lubricant that does not bother the genitals. Keep a clean towel nearby. If there is a phone in the room, turn it off. Try to find a peaceful place free of external noises.

The following exercises will show you how to increase your sensitive concentration. You can practice them with a partner or alone. For the former you will need about an hour and for the latter about thirty minutes.

Celestial touch

1. During this exercise, one member of the pair will play the active part while the other will be passive. One cannot be active and passive at the same time, but the roles can be switched halfway through the exercise.

2. To start out, the woman will be the passive one. She should lie down face up and get comfortable until she is totally relaxed.

3. In the active role, the man must start by softly sliding his hand along the front of her body for about fifteen to twenty minutes. He must touch her slowly and, in this manner, begin stroking her genitals using his fingers or mouth by touching both the inside and outside of the vagina. Use a good deal of lubrication. Concentrate on the areas being touched, and pay special attention to the sensations you are feeling through touch and sight, and become wrapped in these feelings. Remember that right now there are no demands; you are not touching her to give her pleasure or arouse her but to give pleasure to yourself.

4. The only thing the woman must do is remain relaxed and experience the sensations. She should be completely passive with her eyes closed. She should not move or try to respond. She must also not talk unless she is feeling uncomfortable. She need only feel the touch.

5. If the man becomes distracted, he should try to focus back on the part of the body he is caressing. If you notice that her body becomes tense, tap her lightly on the leg to signal her to relax.

6. Try to remain very concentrated and deeply absorbed in touching her, and think about how she feels. If your mind wanders, focus back on the stroking. It doesn't matter how many times you lose concentration, just remember to focus back on the exercise each time it happens.

7. This is a wonderful technique for learning how to relax and connect to your sensations. The only goal is to obtain as much pleasure as possible while the same happens to your partner. If you notice that you are starting to do it mechanically or that you are becoming bored of stroking, switch up the rhythm by trying each time to be slower.

8. Don't start rubbing the clitoris or even try to stimulate it; the exercise is about learning how to control the different stages of arousal.

9. When you have played the active part for about twenty minutes, you may switch to passive. If the both of you wish, you may continue in the same roles for longer.

10. Lie down face up with your legs lightly stretched out in as comfortable a position as possible. Lay your extended arms at your sides or place them behind your head. Once the man has adapted to this position, he should try not to move.

11. The woman will spend the next twenty minutes stroking the front of his body, especially the genitals. She may use her hands, her mouth, or both.

12. The man's job is to focus on how he is being touched and how it feels. He should not move or talk but just let the woman explore the sensation of touching his penis and scrotum.

13. It does not matter if he is erect or not. A flaccid penis should be as attractive to the woman as an erect one. They simply feel different. She will concentrate only on how it feels to touch it not on the arousal of one or both of them. If he is erect, it is important that she understand she does not need to do anything. All that matters to her is enjoying the sensation of seeing him excited.

14. The man should not flex his PC muscle during the exercise. He should also avoid holding his breath. All he needs to do is close his eyes, relax, and concentrate on the touch.

15. If the woman feels the man become tense, she should signal for him to relax by tapping him softly on the leg. The man should only speak if something is making him uncomfortable.

16. If you become distracted, try to refocus your attention on where you are touching him. It does not matter how often your mind wanders; just keep practicing.

17. If you do not have a partner or prefer to practice on your own, sensitive concentration will help you become aware of your body. It is not a technique for masturbation; it is only a way to experience the numerous feelings brought on by arousal. The goal is to create and feel as many sensations as possible.

Alone at last

1. Relax, lie down facing up, and close your eyes. Use plenty of lubrication, and start rubbing yourself slowly and gently. You may wish to begin with the nipples or thighs; both areas are very sensitive. Then move on to the genitals, but stop a while at the stomach, which is also a sensitive area.

2. Once you begin stroking your genitals, do not rub them as you do when masturbating. Do not try to arouse yourself! Explore each crease and fold, and very importantly, take as much time as you need.

3. Remember that the most important thing is to be relaxed and concentrated on the here and now. You are not trying to do anything other than enjoy the sensations. If you are erect, fine; if you are not, that is also okay. You should not purposely try to become erect. There are no goals or demands with this exercise; you should just experience the richness of your own excitement.

4. If your mind wanders, try to gently return to the sensations you are feeling. This may occur several times; it is alright. Simply return your focus to the exercise.

It is good to practice for twenty minutes or longer. Thirty minutes is ideal. At times, the absence of a partner may drive you to rush everything, but this defeats the entire purpose of sensitive concentration. Remember that the emphasis is on sensuality not sexuality.

Increasing the duration of coitus

Increasing the duration of the sexual act is one way of making sure both partners enjoy themselves. There are ways of achieving this and avoiding possible frustration. Put this into practice, and ensure that your sexuality is completely pleasurable.

■ **During sex** the man must breathe abdominally (see page 24). Through the use of deep breathing, one may control the heart rate and then the level of sexual arousal.

■ **When his heart rate** increases and ejaculation is near, the man must interrupt coitus. To regain the initial rhythm, he must withdraw his penis from the vagina, breathe deeply, and hold his breath while clenching his anus muscles hard. He must close his eyes, press his tongue against his palate, and focus his mind. He may also avoid emitting semen by holding the gland of his penis and firmly pressing the frenulum with his thumb. He should not resume sex until the desire to ejaculate has completely vanished.

■ **When ejaculation** is very near, he should put his thumb on the lower part of the penis and squeeze. Another way of controlling ejaculation is by holding the penis with the entire hand and pressing down on the tip with the thumb. Applying pressure in this way reduces the penis's sexual energy and stops the desire to ejaculate.

■ **There is an exercise** that develops the love muscle, which affects the retention of semen. Breathe in while clenching your anus hard until you feel the base of your pelvis lifting and your penis moves. Hold in the air and keep clenching for a few seconds. Exhale and relax. Repeat this exercise several times a day. You may also work this muscle when you use the restroom: clench your anus hard before you are done urinating, thereby cutting off the stream. Hold for a few seconds and relax again. Clench and relax about five times until you have no more urine left, and hold each clench for about ten seconds.

■ **The penetrative technique** used also affects the duration of coitus. Starting from a face to face position, we can see some stark differences. If most of the friction happens between the base of the penis and the clitoris using vertical movement, the female orgasm will happen sooner while the male orgasm is delayed. If, on the other hand, most of the friction happens between the gland of the penis and the walls of the vagina using horizontal movement, it is the male's pleasure that will be heightened.

■ **One position that aids** in the retention of semen is called the fish with overlapping scales (page 79), in which the man lies face up and the woman sits on top of him, causing gravity to exert pressure in the direction opposite than that at which semen will be expelled.

Ascending orgasmic impulse

These techniques are easier to learn after spending four months doing exercises that bolster the vaginal muscles. You will begin learning during the first two weeks without being sexually aroused.

Sit on a chair and breathe abdominally for one minute. Then inhale deeply while clenching your anus and vagina, gritting your teeth, squeezing your fists, and pressing your tongue against your palate. Hold for a few seconds then exhale and relax.

After two weeks are up, continue practicing while sexually aroused. You must hold your breath and clench your muscles once you are approaching orgasm but before vaginal contractions begin.

Mastery of this technique will happen when you notice an intense sensation of heat in the vagina and the rise of sexual energy through the spine. Now you may use this method during sex with your partner.

The orgasm is the most intense experience that a person can feel. It is entirely focused on that person, provides intense pleasure, and is a powerful stimulus to all other senses. Orgasms provide a great deal of energy to the body that we must learn to control.

Submerging yourself in a climax of energy

When a tigress woman is about to have an orgasm, she will direct her energy to her kidneys to stimulate the *Ching* and *Qi*. Then, she will make it rise to her brain in order to experience illumination. Regardless of what she is doing, at the moment of climax she must employ four techniques:

- She places her tongue on her palate to secrete the essence of the red lotus.
- She puts her hands on her ovaries and massages slowly downward.
- She clenches her anus and concentrates on her kidneys.
- She holds her breath during orgasm and exhales when it is over.

According to tradition, after an orgasm tigress women drink the medicine of the Lunar Flower, essence of the lower peak (her own juices), and mixes it with her saliva.

Following this, she will move her tongue in circles around her teeth and gums three times in a clockwise direction and then three more in a counterclockwise direction. She will make the liquid dance over her tongue nine times and will then swallow it only once. With closed eyes, she will feel how it descends to her abdomen.

Erotic massage

There is nothing blander in the world than water,
yet it is only she who may mold even the hardest rock.
In this respect, she is irreplaceable.

During the act of sex, energy is concentrated in the Cinnabar Field, where it bursts during orgasm and then rises to the brain as *Shen*. The even flow of energy in the body is essential for the transformation among the Three Treasures (*Jing*, *Qi*, and *Shen*).

Not only is there an extraordinary burst of *Qi* within the body during coitus, but there is also an exchange of fluids and energy between our body and that of our partner. Good communication between both sexual participants is needed for this transfer to happen.

Massage prepares the body for sex because it bolsters the flow of energy and creates harmony between the two lovers. Thanks to its aphrodisiac-like effects, it may also be used as foreplay.

General techniques

Giving and receiving. Before starting the massage, the couple will decide who is giving and who is receiving. Despite having learned to enjoy touching one another, it is clear that the receiver will benefit the most. Therefore, it is best to exchange roles during the massage. When used as foreplay, it is better for the man to be the last one to give the massage to avoid starting coitus with an imbalance of arousal in the man's favor.

Position. The person receiving the massage lies down on a medium-hard surface (a mat placed on the floor will do), keeps their legs straight and slightly apart, and relaxes all their muscles. To relieve pressure in the vertebrae, it is helpful to place a medium-sized,

The curative power of hands

The hands are one of the energy gates through which *Qi* of the body may interact with the environment. With our hands, we can absorb or project energy to correct imbalances in our bodies or in the body of the person we are massaging.

You are able to feel the energy in the palms of your hands if you hold them about two inches apart. If you hold this position for a few seconds and concentrate, you will feel as though there is a gelatinous substance between them that offers up some resistance when you try to bring your hands together.

There are different ways of using the hands during massage depending on the areas of the body that are being massaged and the goals in mind.

Percussion. Let your closed fists fall on the area you are treating without using force while alternating between both fists as if you were playing a drum. As you let them fall, your fists will bounce up and down on the body while creating vibrations that activate the flow of *Qi*.

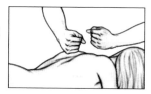

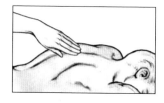

Rubbing with an extended hand. You must keep your fingers extended at all times and exert pressure using the pads at the top of your palm and the base of the fingers. Whoever is performing the massage must press down while dragging the skin forward or backward.

rolled-up towel underneath the neck. The masseuse will take up a comfortable position in which they may reach any part of the receiving participant's body: kneeling or sitting with a straight back and relaxed shoulders.

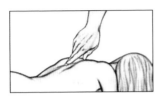

Rubbing with the tips of the fingers. With your fingers extended, use your fingertips to press down and drag the skin.

Pressure using a finger. Press down using the tip of your middle finger with your index finger resting on top of it. This allows for a more useful activation of energy.

Stretching. Form a pincer with your thumb and the rest of your hand as a whole. Keep your fingers together and stretched out. Using this pincer, grab the area you are massaging and stretch the skin using the muscles in your arms.

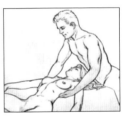

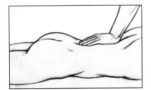

Laying on of hands. Place your stretched-out hands on the desired area, and without moving them, transfer the energy that flows out of them.

Tickling with the fingernails. Lightly graze the surface of the skin using your fingernails. Do not scratch. This will produce a slight tickling sensation.

Circular massage. Move your index and middle fingers in circles on the target area while pressing down. You should use enough strength so that the skin moves with your fingers.

Massage sequence

There are two types of erotic massage: face to face and facing away. In both cases, it is recommended that you begin with the starting phase, which is used to achieve the degree of relaxation necessary for the massage to be effective.

One of the two lovers alone can receive the massage, but in this book we will show a massage sequence in which both members receive the benefits by switching the roles of giver and receiver during the session.

We will begin with the preparatory phase. In this sequence we will do a series of stretches to open our energy gates and ease contact between the couple.

Gate of the Third Eye (the space between the eyebrows). Kneel down beside your partner's head. Gently pinch the skin at the temples using your thumb and index finger and drag it forward. Keep the skin stretched out for one minute. This massage produces an instant relaxing effect and relieves headaches, pain in the eyes, and sinusitis.

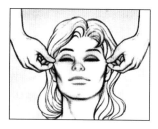

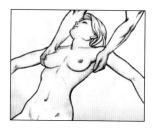

Point 40 Gate (located on both sides of the chest). Form a pincer with your thumb and the rest of your hand, grasp the skin and the sides of the body at chest height, and pull it away from the ribs. Hold it there for one minute. This stretch strengthens breathing and bolsters the immune system because it stimulates the lungs and the thymus gland.

Solar Plexus Gate (at stomach height). Gently hold the skin at the sides of the body at the height of the lower ribs without grasping too hard. In the same way described during the previous stretch, pull it away from the ribs for a minute.

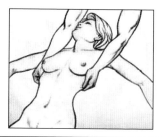

By separating the skin tissue from the ribs, we are easing respiration and relaxing the diaphragm. Doing this will increase oxygenation and the flow of energy inside the body.

Dantian Gate (center of gravity and sexual energy). Pinch the skin at the sides of the body at waist height and stretch it away for a minute. This will relax your partner's Cinnabar Field and get rid of all feelings of fear and guilt, as well as stress.

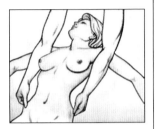

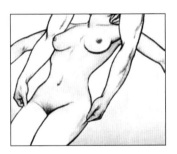

Door of Mortality Gate (perineum). Pinch the skin at the sides of the buttocks where the thighs begin by using your hand as a pincer. Pull it away from the body, like in the previous stretches. You will open the perineum and allow a greater flow of blood and energy in the area of the genitals. Once one of the partners has received this full sequence, it is time to switch roles so that the performer may now receive the benefits of the massage.

In order to properly explain the erotic massage that follows, we will call the person who is receiving frontal massage A and the person who is receiving dorsal massage B. These roles will be switched later, and with practice, each participant will be able to choose the position in which they would rather receive the massage.

We will split the massage into sections, separated by the switching of roles between the giver and the receiver.

Massage sequence

Feeding the Back Door of the Crimson Palace. The receiver of this dorsal massage should lie face down. In this explanation, A will be the giver and B will be the receiver. The giver will execute a laying on of hands on the area between the shoulder blades, known by the name Back Door of the Crimson Palace. This is where tension builds throughout the day due to problems and other disagreeable experiences.

The fingers must be pointing toward the receiver's neck while the hands remain in place for a minute. As your hands are lying in place, you must focus on the energy you are freeing through your palms. Press down deeply and slowly for a few seconds and then gradually let up as if there were glue between your hands and your partner's body.

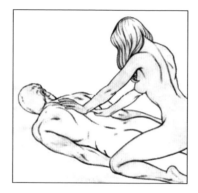

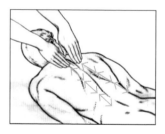

Strengthening the spine. Beginning at the seventh cervical vertebra, found in the neck bone that sticks out, start massaging using the tips of your fingers. Place your fingers over the specified area and press forward and backward while, moving downward toward the sacrum. The massage should be rhythmic and make the receiver's body vibrate. This normally takes about thirty seconds but may last a little longer if you lack practice. Once you have arrived at the sacrum, repeat the massage. This part of the massage helps eliminate back pain caused by poor posture. It is important to place your hands on either side of the backbone.

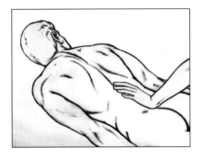

Feeding the Gate of the Backbone. The massage moves on with a laying on of hands upon the sacrum, or Gate of the Backbone, for one minute with fingers pointing toward the neck. This area helps with feelings of security, curing sexual trauma, and relieving sciatic and lumbar pain, weakness of the legs, and problems of the prostate and uterus.

Opening of the Gate of the Backbone. This part of the massage has effects similar to those before and is used as a complement. Place yourself between your partner's legs, and place your hands on each side of the sacrum with your thumbs perpendicular to the rest of your fingers and pointing at each other. The rest of your fingers should point toward the neck. Press down lightly with the right thumb while dragging it up about two inches (taking about two seconds), and then repeat with the left thumb. Repeat, alternating between both thumbs, for a minute.

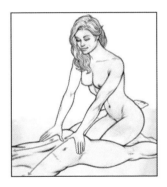

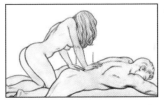

Ascension of energy through the backbone. The purpose here is to make energy flow from the sacrum up to the crown through the governing vessel. Remain situated between your partner's legs, and place one hand over the sacrum. Press forward with your palm (refer to the massage technique using an extended hand), and place the other one just where

Massage sequence

the first ends. The laying on of one hand must immediately follow the lifting of the previous hand. Ascend, hand over hand, toward the crown. Go slowly, and focus on the flow of energy inside your partner's body and through your hands.

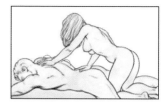

Relaxing the back muscles. Kneel down beside your partner's head. Place your hands on both sides of the backbone at neck height, and begin the descent toward the sacrum. Use the same technique as before while keeping your hands at the same height. You should touch the muscles around the backbone not the backbone itself. Upon reaching the sacrum, direct your hands toward each hip and move back up along the sides of the torso towards the shoulders. Next, move your hands back to the bone behind the neck where the massage began. Repeat the entire cycle for about three minutes (seven cycles).

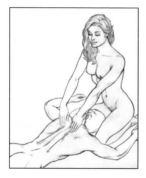
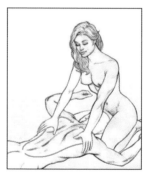

Percussion on the Back Door of the Crimson Palace. Perform a percussion massage (see page 108) by letting your fists fall on the area between the shoulder blades. You should exert no additional pressure; the force of

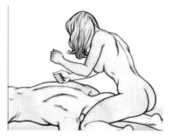

gravity is enough. Let one fist fall first, then the other, while maintaining a constant rhythm for a minute.

This massage increases one's mood and relieves tachycardia, palpitations, asthma, emphysema, anxiety, and insomnia.

Percussion on the Gate of the Backbone. You should not perform this massage if your partner is suffering from any back injuries. Place yourself between your partner's legs and rhythmically massage the sacrum using the percussion method. Continue for one minute. This technique helps address poor circulation in the legs, paralysis of the lower limbs, impotence, vaginitis, urinary problems, and lumbago.

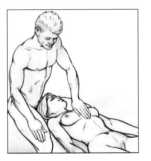

Feeding the Crimson Palace. During these massages, we will switch so that B will be the giver and A the receiver. These are frontal massages during which A will lie face up. Place one hand over the sternum, fingers pointing toward the feet, and gently press downward. This massage fights depression and introversion and increases confidence and understanding between the couple.

Toning the internal organs. Kneel down next to your partner, and place your hands over the ribs about halfway between the chest and the belly button. Use the palms of your hands to rub in a crosswise direction slowly and with light pressure for three minutes.

This technique helps with digestion and the production of blood in the vicinity of the spleen.

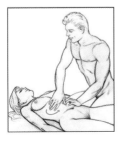

Massage sequence

Feeding the Solar Plexus (upper abdomen). Use the laying on of hands method on the upper abdomen with fingers pointed downward. Keep your hand on this area for thirty seconds. Using this massage will invigorate the nervous system and relax your partner's diaphragm.

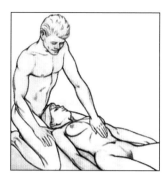

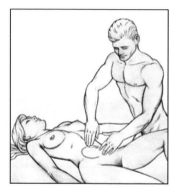

Toning the dantian (lower abdomen, sexual energy center). Rub your hands to warm them up and, once they are hot, make circles using your fingertips around the belly button while stroking your partner's skin. Make complete circles with both hands at the same time in the same direction. Move one hand over the other when they cross each other's paths.

This toning massage activates sexual desire and relieves anxiety, constipation, menstrual pains, and headaches.

Feeding the dantian. Use the laying on of hands technique on your partner's lower abdomen with fingers pointing downward for thirty seconds.

This will stimulate the flow of energy and generate confidence and a sense of security for both partners.

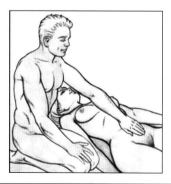

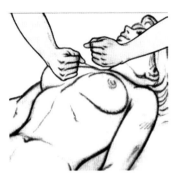

Percussion on the Crimson Palace. Kneel down next to your partner's head and perform a rhythmic percussion on their sternum for a minute. If the woman is receiving the massage, limit the percussion to the area between the breasts to avoid hitting them.

Doing this massage will ignite your partner's passion, as well as regulating their respiratory functions and relieving muscular tension in the chest area.

Channeling energy toward the dantian. Place your hands on the sternum with your fingers pointing downward. Drag your hands toward the pubis using the rubbing with an extended hand technique. When you arrive at the lower abdomen, separate your hands and drag them toward the hips. Then move them up along the sides of the torso until reaching the underarms and bring them back together at the sternum. Repeat this cycle for five minutes with each cycle lasting about thirty seconds.

This technique increases confidence in people who are afraid of sexual relationships. It also prepares the body for coitus.

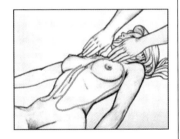

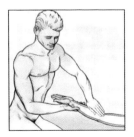

Tickling the arms. Take your partner's hand palm up and massage by dragging your fingernails along the inside of the arm up to the underarm. Descend along the outside of the arm until arriving back at the wrist.

This massage will awaken your partner's passion. The tickling on the arm is very stimulating, and the receiver will feel ripples of energy through the throat and bellow the belly.

Massage sequence

Pinching the underarm. Place your thumb in the center of your partner's underarm and the rest of your fingers on their pectoral muscles. Exert pressure in a circular pattern with the thumb inside the underarm and the rest of the fingers on the pectoral muscle. This technique must follow the previous one because it relaxes and relieves tension after the buildup of excitement from the tickling massage.

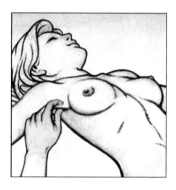

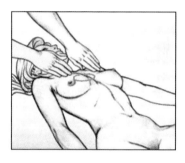

Opening of the Door of the Crimson Palace. Place your hand on the sternum, and massage using a circular motion with the tips of your fingers for about thirty seconds. The technique of the Opening of the Door of the Crimson Palace strengthens confidence, happiness, and one's mood.

Channeling energy toward the perineum. Let's switch roles again. The following are dorsal massages. A will give, and B will receive. Place yourself on your knees next to your partner's head. Your partner will be lying face down. Starting at the neck, softly drag your fingernails down along both sides of the backbone and over the buttocks until reaching the perineum (between the anus and sexual organs).

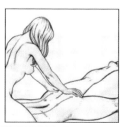
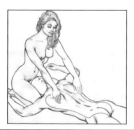

Using your middle finger, press down on the center of the perineum for a few seconds. Continue back up, tickling the sides of the torso until reaching the shoulders, and bring your hands together at the neck. If your partner cannot stand the tickling, you can replace the technique with an extended hand massage. The therapeutic goals of this massage consist of eliminating fear and anxiety by properly channeling energy.

Opening of the perineum. Kneel down next to your partner's head, and place your hands on the lower section of their buttocks next to the thighs. Push them lightly upward and downward for about thirty seconds.

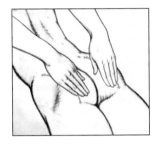

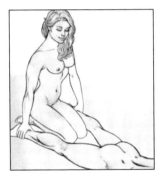

Holding the ankles. Get down on your knees at the bottom of your partner's legs and hold the ankles with your palms on each foot's instep. Next, twist your partner's feet inward. Hold this position for about thirty seconds. This technique increases the body's strength and bolsters the brain and eyes.

Ascension of energy through the legs. Start at the previous position, and move your fingernails over your partner's skin going up along the inside of their thighs until reaching the buttocks. Keep going up over the buttocks until reaching the hips, and come back down along the outside of the legs until arriving at the ankles. Do this five times.

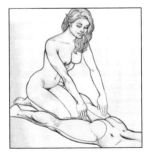

Massage sequence

Buttocks massage. Starting at the ankles, move upward to the buttocks using an extended hand massage technique. Once there, stroke the perineum with your fingertips. Keep moving upward, over the anus, to the top of the buttocks, and then back down in a circle.

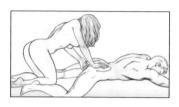

Keep massaging with extended hands until you go over the whole buttocks and arrive back at the perineum, where you will resume massaging with your fingertips. Repeat this entire sequence for three minutes.

Opening of the Gate of Mortality. Place your thumbs on the perineum and the rest of your hands on the buttocks. Press down using circular motions with your thumbs on the perineum and the rest of your hands on the buttocks.

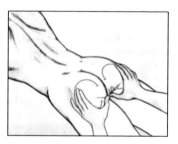

Channeling sexual energy. We are going to switch roles again. B will be giving, and A will be receiving the frontal massage. Kneel down next to your partner's head, and beginning at the sternum, stroke the skin with your fingernails. Move down to the pubis, work around it, and keep going until you reach the perineum. Press the center of the perineum using your middle finger and then continue dragging your fingernails toward the hips. Move up along the sides of the torso until your hands meet again at the sternum while lightly brushing the nipples along the way. Repeat this cycle for three minutes.

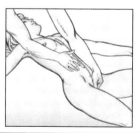
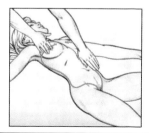

Holding the ankles. Place yourself between your partner's legs, and hold the back of their ankles hard for thirty seconds. This technique awakens an enjoyable feeling of confidence. Holding the ankles is the beginning to the following exercises, which will consist of cycles of tickling the legs. They are very sexually stimulating.

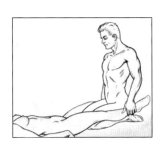

Cycling along the calves. Begin at the ankles and move upward along the inside of the calves until reaching the knees. Move back down along the outside

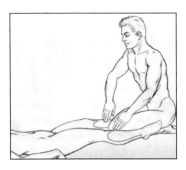

while softly dragging your fingernails along your partner's skin. In this case, you may use your fingertips in place of your fingernails. The goal of this technique is to trigger the sensitivity of the desired area using light tickling. Repeat this cycle for one minute.

This technique tends to be very pleasurable because it causes a heightened level of arousal for the recipient, which makes it very useful for motivating your partner when it comes time to have sex.

Cycling along the thighs. Start at the knees and move up along the lower part of the thighs until reaching the groin. Keep moving toward the hips and then back down along the outside while dragging your fingernails along your partner's skin. This massage should be done immediately after cycling along the calves. This will raise the recipient's level of arousal.

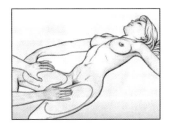

Sequence of sensual massage in the mind

These movements are relaxing and very enjoyable for the man as much as the woman. They are: (1) "Watering the kidneys": massage the ears, known as the outer flowers of the kidneys, until they become warm. (2) "Knocking on the door".

(3) "The path of the eyes": the right eye is connected to the energy of the Sun (*Yang*) and the left eye to the Moon (*Yin*). (4) "Feeding the cheeks", or the "Middle warmer". (5) "Strengthening good will", or energy of the kidneys. (6) "Disciplining the emotions": the jaw area may store rage or resentment. (7) "Erasing the mask". (8 and 9) "Opening the door". And finally, (10) the "final resting" position.

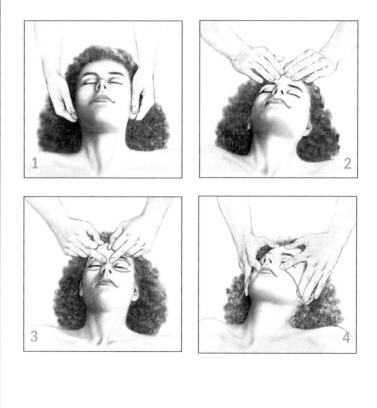

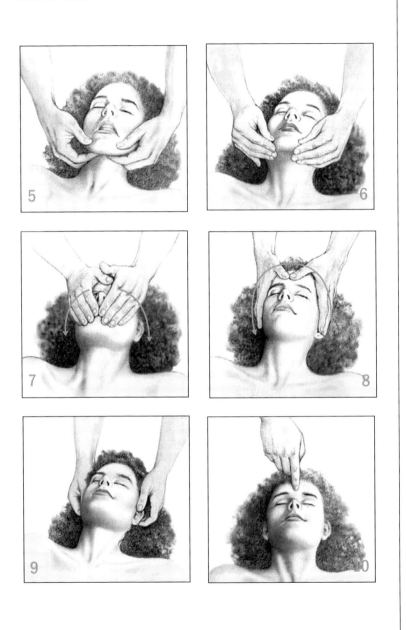

Sexual massage

Until now, the massages we have been practicing have been used to prepare the body for the act of love without focusing on the sexual organs. They stimulate the flow of energy through the body and concentrate it in the sexual organs. The following massages stimulate the genitals and produce intense pleasure for both the giver and the recipient.

It is preferable that the woman be the recipient of these massages. It is only recommendable to perform them on the man if he does not have an erection. This way, we may avoid premature ejaculation.

Hair pulling. Superficially caress the pubic hair, and after a few seconds, take small handfuls and gently tug on them. Start at the top of the pubis and travel downward, bit by bit until reaching the vulva.

Cycling around the labia minora

Using your fingertips, stroke the inner part of your partner's thighs until reaching the perineum. From there, continue along the inner crease of one labia minora (between the labia minora, the vaginal opening, and urethra) until reaching the clitoris. Massage the skin that covers it in a circular motion, and descend down the outer crease (between the labia majora and minora) until reaching the perineum. Repeat the cycle going around the opposite labia minora. Remember that at all times the massage must be slow and soft without excessive force.

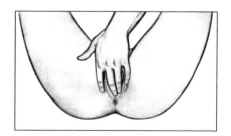

Pulling skin. Stroke the inner thighs and groin. Separate the outer labia and, using the index finger and thumb, pinch some of the skin and gently pull it upwards. Let it go at the last second. Start near the vaginal opening and keep going along the outer labia, and finish near the clitoris. Do this about six times.

Repeat the massage along the opposite outer labia and then along both labia at the same time using both hands. Repeat the entire massage along the inner labia while always finishing at the skin covering the clitoris.

Circling over the clitoris

Use the tip of your index finger to rub the skin covering the clitoris in a clockwise direction and then in the opposite direction. Do about twelve circles in each direction, varying the amount of pressure at random. Next, place your middle finger under the clitoris so that the hood covering it rests above your finger. Rhythmically move the finger up and down while covering and uncovering the clitoris as you drag the skin along. You must use light pressure during this massage. Remember that it is very important to be completely relaxed during this massage in order to find the clitoris. If there is no lubrication, you will not be able to drag the skin back to uncover the clitoris. Continue with the vertical movements along the clitoris and the skin while lightly increasing the pressure and the rhythm.

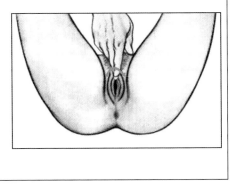

Stroking the vaginal opening. Move the tip of your middle finger in a circle around the vaginal opening. Next, gently introduce the finger into the vagina and exert pressure on the opening as you remove it. Practice inserting and withdrawing the finger while applying pressure to a different part of the vagina each time.

Opening the tripod. Press down on the center of the perineum using your pinky finger, and insert your index, middle, and ring finger in the vagina up to the third phalange. While pressing the perineum, separate your three fingers and press them up against the walls of the vagina. Keep applying pressure for a few seconds and then relax. Repeat this cycle ten times.

Removing the honey. Insert your middle finger deep into the vagina and move it in clockwise circles while pressing the walls of the vagina. You can place your thumb on the clitoris, but keep your fingernail from touching and possibly harming it. Next, keep massaging in circles going the opposite direction. Make ten circles in each direction.

Pressing the G-spot. During this massage, we will locate the woman's famous pleasure point: the G-spot. Insert your middle finger up to the first phalange and rub it against the anterior wall of the vagina (behind which is the bladder). Move it up and down using minimal displacement and applying deep pressure for three minutes.

Caressing the pubic hair. The following massages are for men. Stroke the pubic hair on your partner's testicles, penis, and perineum. Take small handfuls, starting at the belly button and moving down to the scrotum, and tug them gently.

Cycling over the inner penis

If there is no erection, hold the gland of the penis with one hand, lift it, and rest the back of your hand on his belly. With your other hand, lift the scrotum up, hold that position for a few seconds to transfer heat to the area, and then release your hand from the scrotum. Next, using the thumb of the hand that was holding the scrotum, drag down on the skin of the penis until you touch your other hand. Hold the penis with both your hands and warm it. Keep holding the gland with one hand, and with the other, gently stroke the penis by descending down the middle, passing over the scrotum, and arriving at the perineum. Then, press down on the perineum for a few seconds using your middle finger. Repeat the cycle for a couple of minutes until there is an erection.

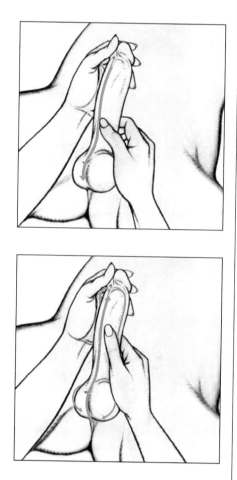

If he is already erect, hold the gland in the same way with one hand with the back of the hand facing his belly. With your other hand's thumb, softly caress the perineum and move upward, along the scrotum and the middle of the penis until reaching the gland. Slowly move back down along the sides of the penis and scrotum until returning to the perineum. Repeat this cycle for two minutes.

Massaging the gland

If there is no erection, lean his penis against his belly while holding it with your hand between his abdomen and his penis. Use your other hand's thumb to massage the penis from the bottom up. Once you reach the gland, massage the frenulum (the flap of skin connecting the foreskin to the gland) with circular movements for about a minute.

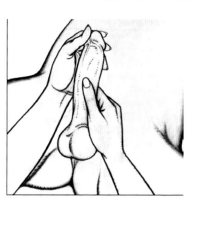

If he is already erect, hold the gland with one hand and pull down the foreskin. Using your other hand's index finger and thumb, form a circle around the penis just under the gland and rotate it in both directions. Do this for a minute while applying constant light pressure. In the case of someone who ejaculates prematurely, it is best to skip this massage.

Other massages for men. The following massages are to be done once the man is erect but never in the case of someone who ejaculates prematurely. If you are planning on having sex after the massage, it will be necessary to wait for a little while so the man may become less aroused. During this time, he should perform sexual massage on the woman.

■ **The countdown.** Wrap your right hand around the upper part of the penis, and hold the testicles with your left hand with fingers pointing toward the perineum. This massage is made up of two movements. During the first, you must lower your right hand, dragging it down the penis while lifting the scrotum upward with your left hand. During the second movement, you must raise your right hand back up while lowering your left, which is the opposite of the first movement. Do the first movement ten times to begin with followed by ten of the second movement. Continue with nine of the first followed by nine of the second, then eight and eight, etc.

■ **Squeezing.** Hold the penis with one hand, and place the palm of the other hand on top of the gland. Press down on the gland while twisting the hand in both directions like squeezing the juice out of an orange. Do this about twenty times.

■ **Working in sequence.** Cover the gland with one hand, and drag it down so that the gland emerges at the top through the ring formed by the thumb and index finger. Place your other hand over the gland and drag it down, as well. You must keep the gland from completely emerging, so work quickly. Keep placing one hand behind the other, covering the gland, and keeping up a constant rhythm.

Enjoying sex with acupressure

Bend down and you shall be straight.
Empty yourself and you shall be full.
Decay and you shall renew.
Wish and you shall receive.

Acupressure, or shiatsu, is a Chinese medicinal technique that corrects imbalances of energy that cause illness. It consists of using the fingers to apply pressure to certain points called meridians, which are the channels through which energy flows in the body. It is used to treat illnesses and alleviate pain.

Acupuncture acts on the same points as acupressure. The difference, however, is that acupuncture uses needles instead of fingers and requires greater precision.

General technique

Participants during massage. The participants present during massage are the masseuse or practitioner (the person giving the massage) and the patient, who is the recipient.

In our case, the acupressure will take place between a couple, so the roles of the giver and the recipient will depend on the chosen treatment. For example, if we wish to treat a case of premature ejaculation, the woman will take on the role of the masseuse, and the man will be the patient.

Preparing. Energy flows throughout our whole bodies. When we apply pressure to a specific point, we are awakening that vital energy present in each one of our organs. The attitude of the person performing the massage is of great importance. They must be relaxed, calm, and full of love because their disposition will be transferred to their partner. When treating against impotence and frigidity, it is essential that the masseuse be in top physical and spiritual condition and, most importantly, believe in what they are doing. It is this energy that they will be transferring to their partner.

When using acupressure for erotic stimulation or to treat against exhaustion, you must not forget that the performer's attitude must be harmonious so that their *Yang* energy may complement with tranquility or the patient's *Yin* energy.

The following box shows you the secrets behind doing each massage correctly.

How to proceed

MASSEUSE

- We recommend massaging with naked arms or with a complete lack of clothing to facilitate movement.
- Hands should be well taken care of with fingernails rounded using limestone.
- The masseuse must wash their hands with soap and water, alcohol, or cologne before and after each massage session.
- The performer must harmonize the work of both hands, which correspond with *Yin* and *Yang*, in order to maintain balance. They must also identify themselves through their hands. This is the true secret of massage—the door that permits entrance into the dominion of the art of acupressure. This state may only be achieved with practice. Your skills as a masseuse will improve considerably given enough time.

PATIENT

- The patient rests comfortably on a massage table that may be accessed by either side.

ENJOYING SEX WITH ACUPRESSURE

> - It is better to be naked in order to ease the location and manipulation of the points to be treated. Any areas that will not immediately be treated may be covered with a towel.
> - When the patient lies faceup, they will place a pillow under their head to keep it slightly elevated. They will place two more pillows under the popliteal fossa (the space behind the knees) of each leg in order to achieve complete muscular relaxation.
> - When the patient lies face down, their body will relax on the flat surface of the table with their forehead sitting on the forearm and ankles slightly elevated with the help of a pillow.

What to use to apply pressure. Your hands are your most valuable tool for massaging. Take full advantage of the soft and supple parts, such as the tips of the fingers. They must be warm so that when you apply pressure to the patient, they feel pleasure and do not notice a change in temperature. If you have cold hands, the sensation may not be enjoyable. In the following paragraph, you will find a brief description of the different parts of the hand that are used for acupressure.

- **The thumb.** You should apply pressure using the part of the tip closest to the joint of the first phalange and not with the top of the finger. This way you can apply more pressure with less effort.

- **Index, middle, and ring fingers.** Apply pressure with the tips. These fingers are used to treat the points on the ankle, the face, and the abdomen.

- **Palm of the hand.** It applies pressure to the eyes and the abdomen. The palms are used for vibratory massages and for massaging the tendons and extenders of the ankle.

How to apply pressure

Pressure must be intense but not painful. The force necessary to apply pressure comes from the weight of the masseuse herself, not from the arm muscles. The masseuse will let her body weight push her hands as she is massaging.

Massage techniques

BRUSHING MASSAGE (USING THE FINGERTIPS)

Done using the fingertips. It must be very soft like a caress.

FRICTION MASSAGE (USING THE WHOLE HAND)

You must hold the area to be treated in your hands while squeezing firmly and transferring heat.

DEEP MASSAGE (USING THE PALMS OF THE HAND)

Applied using the palms of the hand by dragging them forcefully along the desired surface.

PRESSURE MASSAGE

The part of the hand that applies pressure, intensity, length, and direction varies in each case:

- The intensity of the pressure may be light, like a caress, or strong, shaving away the pain.
- The hand will take on different shapes for the massage, according to the needs of the target area, whether it be flat or round, bony or muscular, etc.

When pressure must be applied to a less muscular area, you will use your fingertips (the part behind the joint that joins the first and second phalanges) to knead the area to be treated.

Sometimes we may use the heel of the hand to massage a round bodily surface covered with a thick muscular cloak.

In some cases, pressure is applied using all fingers, as well as the palm of the hand. Other times, only the middle and index fingers are used, or even just the thumb while using the rest of the hand to brace the desired area. When it is necessary to be soft and precise, pressure will be continuous and usually digital.

Generally, pressure is applied from the periphery toward the center. In other words, it follows the circulatory system, stimulating the flow of energy. In some cases, however, it may be applied in the opposite direction. When the pressure must be applied to a specific muscle, it is advantageous to follow the grain of the muscle fibers.

- **Pinching massage.** This massage is done by pinching and squeezing the desired area between the thumb and index finger. Pinching pressure, when executed correctly, is not painful. It is only uncomfortable when applied roughly or too hard. This technique tends to be applied on smaller surfaces in the abdominal region. It stimulates organic exchanges in the treated area and causes the expulsion of undesired buildups.

- **Holding massage.** Apply pressure with your thumb on the desired point while holding the area with the rest of the hand. As long as you continue to apply pressure, you must retain contact between your fingers and the area you are treating. It is recommendable to combine pressure and distention to stimulate the pumping of energy.

- **Pincer massage.** Similar to the pinching massage except it must be smoother, more delicate, and generally more prolonged.

- **Circular massage.** Move your index and middle fingers in circles on the target area while pressing down. You should use enough strength so that the skin moves with your fingers.

How to know if the pressure is adequate. We must communicate constantly with our patient in order to gauge the effectiveness of our acupressure. They will let us know if energy is flowing correctly. The first thing they will feel is a small rippling, tickles, or a numbness in the treated area. At the same time, they may feel their body temperature rising, although this is not always the case.

The patient may also feel the effects of the applied pressure spreading to other parts of the body. This is a natural reaction, especially during sessions that stimulate points connected with the genitals.

Another way of knowing if we are applying pressure correctly is by observing the point we are massaging. If we feel a change in the tissues under the skin, this is an unmistakable sign that energy is flowing through the whole body.

Length of the massage. The length of the massage depends on the number of points we are treating. However, it is safe to say that none of the treatments described in this chapter are excessively long. For the most part, none of them spend more than five minutes on a single point.

Remember that it is convenient to pause in between each press. It is also beneficial to preface each massage by brushing or rubbing the areas adjacent to the point in question so that energy may flow more easily.

How to find the points. A pressure point occupies a very small area on the human body and may be very hard to find for someone who has not practiced. However, by measuring the distances from certain reference points, such as the belly button, the ankle bone, the nipples, etc., it is easier to find the exact location of the point in question.

We will be using units of measurement that are not universal. That is to say, they will vary from person to person. In each case, the unit will be proportional to the recipient's body.

In acupressure, the word unit refers to the width of the thumb of the person receiving the massage, or the patient. For example, if we say that point 8 is three units under the belly button, it means that it is three times the width of the patient's thumb away from the belly button.

It is easier for the recipient him- or herself to locate the points, but if the masseuse wishes to make the measurement, they must compare the width of their thumb with the patient's before beginning.

Now you are ready to begin massaging. When you become familiar with each one of the points used in acupressure and how to locate them, it will be easier to use each treatment that makes use of these methods. Don't forget that you must be relaxed in order to transfer your serenity on to your partner. It is very important that you take your time and follow the guidelines described at the beginning of the chapter. You must also keep in mind a few precautionary rules. Acupressure is not advisable in the following cases:

- During **pregnancy**, no pressure should be applied to the side of the abdomen or the lower back to avoid hurting the fetus or causing a miscarriage.

- During the presence of **infectious illnesses**, bacterial or viral, in order to avoid spreading them.

- When there is a high **fever**, which is a sign of internal infection.

- If there are **pimples** or **boils** on the area to be treated as they may become infected. However, massage can be beneficial for areas of the skin affected by acne, eczema, or psoriasis.

- In the presence of **inflammatory diseases**, such as thrombophlebitis or painful varicose veins, because the pressure on these areas may increase the discomfort.

- When there are **open wounds, scabs, or recent surgery**. It is better not to manipulate these areas in order to avoid delaying the healing process.

- When there are strange **lumps** or pain in the area we wish to treat.

- **After eating** to avoid interrupting digestion. It is recommendable to wait two hours after eating a meal and to avoid eating during the massage.

Acupressure points

There are two kinds of points: individual and double points. Double points are those that actually consist of two points that exist symmetrically along the vertical axis of the body. Individual points exist by themselves whether it is because they are located on top of the vertical axis or because they connect to a meridian that is only found on one side of the body.

When using a double point, pressure must be applied to both halves of the double point. This necessitates the use of both hands. The length of the pressure indicated by the instructions should not be halved.

Point 1. Located on the soles of the feet, it is considered a double point. To find it, you must bend your toes until forming a horizontal line on the bottom of the foot. Then, use both hands to squeeze the sides of the foot until you see a vertical line. The point is located at the intersection of both lines. This point affects the dispersal of energy and is directly connected to the suprarenal glands. This massage is

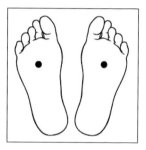

traditionally used to treat people who are faced with feelings of fear or inhibition before sex. It also helps fight cystitis, dysmenorrhea, and urinary incontinence. Stimulating this point also vigorously stimulates the sexual organs and the immune system.

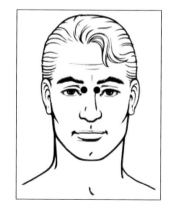

Point 2. This double point is located next to the eyes between the nose and tear ducts. It is directly connected to the fifth toe on the foot and affects the kidneys. It is used to treat certain ocular diseases, as well as cephalalgia and any other kind of headache. This point is used during acupressure to cure dizziness. It is used during acupuncture to treat conjunctivitis, sinusitis, and rhinitis.

Point 3. Double point found on the back of the hand at the junction between the first and second metacarpals, which are the five bones that connect to the finger bones in the hand. To find the points, we must separate the thumb and index finger. This is one of the most well-known and used points due to its sedative and relaxing effects. It is especially useful before starting acupressure massage to carefully press these two points for a few minutes. This will create an excellent balance of energy in the entire body. It is also interesting to apply pressure to the point when your patient is suffering from headaches, toothaches, or other rheumatic problems in the arms and shoulders. It aids in the absorption and elimination of heavy residues.

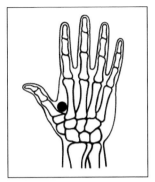

Point 4. Double point located in the center of the palm that forms part of the Sexuality Circulation meridian, which begins at the thorax two units above the nipple and runs down the arm until reaching the top of the middle finger. The point is connected to the heart, circulation, and sex organs. Massaging this point is very stimulating for the recipient, especially if they are fatigued. It may also tone the body, activate blood circulation, and create an enjoyable sensation of rest and tranquility.

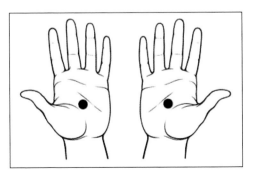

Acupressure points

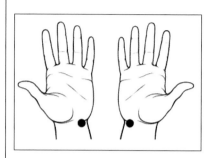

Point 5. Double point found in the crease of the wrist in line with the pinky finger in a small hole formed when we bend the fist down. Acupressure on this point is used to fight *Yin* states (depression, general lethargy, fear, inhibitions...), and using acupuncture here helps with vertigo.

Point 6. Double point situated two units below the crease of the wrist between two of the tendons in the forearm. This is one of the most important acupressure points and is used to address impotence or frigidity. It may also be used to treat vomiting, amnesia, insomnia, and insecurity.

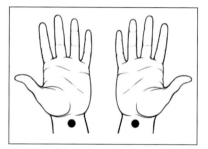

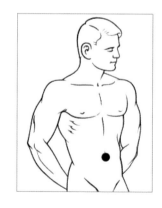

Point 7. Individual point located on the belly one unit below the belly button on top of the body's vertical axis. Massaging it is very beneficial for tired patients and may be used as a complement to weight loss cures, as well as treating insomnia and impotence.

Point 8. Individual point located on the belly three units below the belly button on top of the body's vertical axis. This point is closely related to point 7. Its effects are very similar, but this point may also be used to calm feelings of fear.

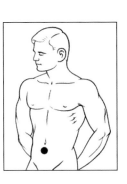

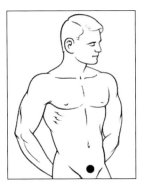

Point 9. Individual point located on the belly four units below the belly button on top of the body's vertical axis. This is the lowest point of all the ones mentioned so far. Its effects are similar to the previous two, and it is particularly effective for treating exhaustion.

Point 10. Individual point located in the center of the perineum at equal distance between the genitals and the anus. It is closely linked to the central nervous system. This point is in the same spot for both men and women. Massaging it is very useful in cases of impotence, fear, and disquiet. In acupuncture, point 10 is usually chosen to fight illnesses such as urethritis, diarrhea, and amenorrhea.

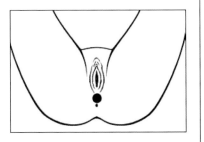

Acupressure points

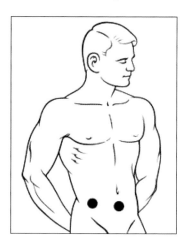

Point 11. Double point located on the belly two units away from the vertical axis on each side at the same height as point 7. This point is used during acupressure to sexually stimulate the recipient of the massage. It is ideal for people experiencing lack of appetite or loss of energy.

Point 12. Double point located on the belly two units away from the vertical axis on each side at the same height as point 9. Its effects are similar to those of point 11. During acupuncture, this point is used to treat illnesses of the male and female sexual organs.

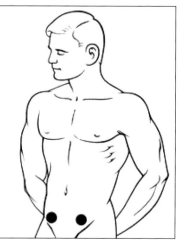

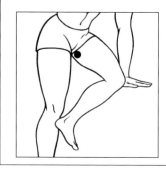

Point 13. Double point found on the inner thigh two units below the crease at the groin. This point is used during acupressure to effectively fight against fear. It is very important in the case of female patients, as it is very useful for treating problems like frigidity.

Point 14. Double point located in the area where the thigh meets the knee on top of the kneecap. Its effects are similar to those of the previous point, and it is used to treat pain in the ovaries.

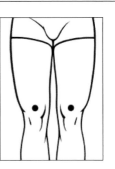

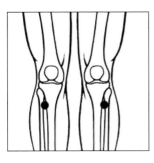

Point 15. Double point that is situated in the hole just beneath the top of the tibia in between the tibia and fibula. It is the most utilized point in acupuncture due to its strong energetic reactions in the core of the body. During acupressure, it is used to fight states of depression, exhaustion, and hypertension (lower tension).

Point 16. Double point located three units below the knee and half a unit toward the outside of the leg (starting at the vertical axis running up the center of the front of the leg) between the tibia and fibula—about three units away from point 15.

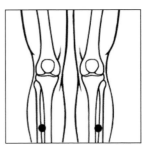

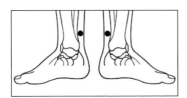

Point 17. Double point found three units above the inner ankle bone on the back edge of the tibia. It is very effective at treating female genital diseases.

Acupressure points

Point 18. Double point located in the middle of the horizontal line that links the inner ankle bone with the Achilles tendon. One can feel a soft pulsating in this point. It is particularly useful when the patient is tired, weak, or suffering from spasms.

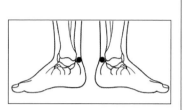

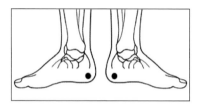

Point 19. Double point situated in the hole found about two units under the inner ankle bone. Its effects are similar to those of the previous point. It is also used for diminishing menstrual pains.

Point 20. Double point located on the back of the foot between the first and second metatarsals, the five bones that are connected to the toes, and two units away from the webbing. During acupuncture, this point is used to treat ocular, nasal, auditory, and rheumatic diseases. It is also useful in the treatment of dysmenorrhea.

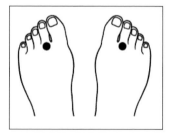

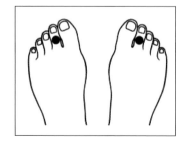

Point 21. Double point located just next to the outer corner of the nail on the second toe. Acupuncture uses this point to calm nerves, get rid of nightmares, and relieve rheumatic pain.

Point 22. Double point located three units away from the vertical axis of the backbone on the horizontal line between the second and third vertebrae (on the upper part of the shoulder blades). This is a special point for treating anemia since stimulating it increases the production of red blood cells.

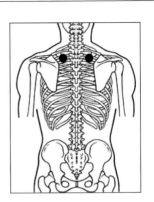

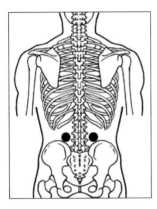

Point 23. Double point located at the back one and a half units away from the vertical axis of the backbone on the horizontal line that passes through the belly button between the second and third lumbar vertebrae. Stimulating this point through the use of acupressure serves to relieve stomach aches.

Point 24. Double point found on the back three units away from the vertical axis of the backbone at the same height as the previous point, about belly button height. Treating this point is very important for men. It allows for better ejaculation control, which increases sexual pleasure.

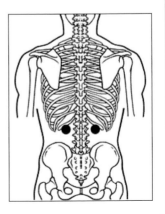

Acupressure points

Point 25. Individual point located on the back on the vertical axis of the backbone between the third and fourth lumbar vertebrae. Treating this point is important for mature women, as it helps with the upsets caused by menopause.

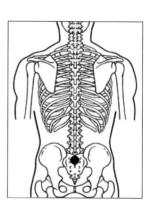

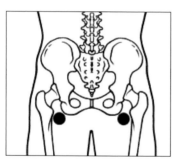

Point 26. Double point located at the lower back one and a half units away from the vertical axis on a horizontal line below the fifth lumbar vertebra.

Points 27, 28, 29, and 30. Point 27 is a double point located on the lower back in the first hole of the sacrococcygeus bone. The next double point, 28, is in the second hole of the sacrococcygeus bone. Double point 29 is in the third hole. Lastly, double point 30 is located in the fourth hole of the sacrococcygeus bone. Acupressure uses these points to treat female frigidity and to bring passion back to a sexually unmotivated couple.

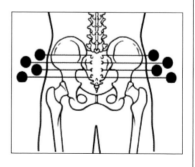

Point 31. Individual point found on top of the backbone between the neck and shoulder blades. It is useful in treating cases of depression and nervousness.

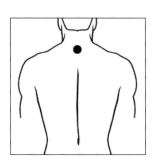

Point 32. Double point located half a unit below the middle of the line that joins the inner ankle bone with the small toe on the inner arch of the foot. Acupressure makes use of this point to treat states of depression and neuralgia.

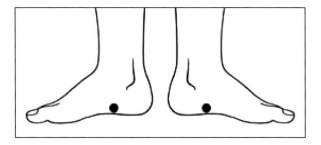

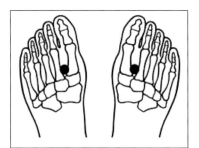

Point 33. Double point found on the back of the foot where the first and second metatarsals (the five bones that are connected to the toes) join under the protuberance of the scaphoid bones and about two units away from point 20. It is used to control the male spirit.

Acupressure points

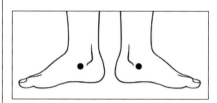

Point 34. Double point found one unit away from the ankle along the middle of the line that connects the inner ankle bone with the small toe. You can find it by starting at the highest point of curvature of the bridge and moving upward one unit.

Point 35. Double point located on the back of the foot between the fourth and fifth metatarsals two units away from the webbing.

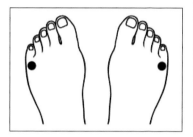

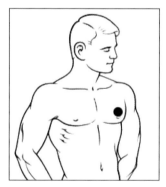

Point 36. Individual point that is unique to men. Located one unit above the right nipple. Massaging this point relieves sharp pains and tones the male genitals.

Point 37. Double point that lies on the outer edge of the hand in line with the pinky one unit away from the pisiform bone. You may find it by starting at point 5 and moving one unit toward the pinky. It is used to treat states of nervousness.

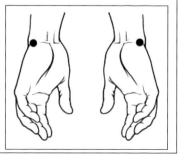

Point 38. Double point located four units above each nipple. Stimulating this point is very calming, and in acupuncture it is used to relieve asthma attacks and other respiratory problems.

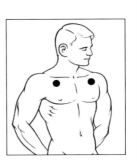

Point 39. Double point found one unit below the outer ankle bone at the height of the fifth toe. It is very important for the treatment of cystitis and dysmenorrhea.

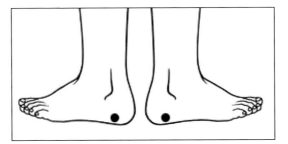

Point 40. Individual point found in the center of the chest just where the breasts begin. It is used to treat all manners of genitourinary diseases, as well as asthma and other respiratory diseases.

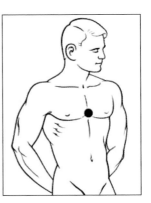

Acupressure points

Point 41. Double point located on the back of the shoulder between the clavicle and shoulder blade. It is normally used to treat rheumatic diseases and shoulder pains. Acupressure also uses it for its sedative effects in cases of hypertension and anxiety.

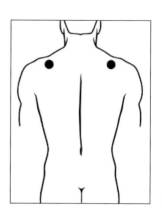

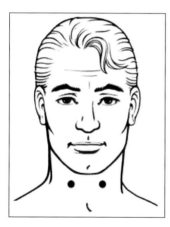

Point 42. Double point found on the neck on both sides of the larynx and below the jaw. Stimulating this point amplifies the orgasm and relieves emotional stress and fatigue that affects sexual performance.

Point 43. Individual point situated between the upper lip and the nose. In the woman's case, it is connected to the clitoris, and massaging this point stimulates vital energy and amplifies orgasm. In the man's case, stimulating this point helps to control ejaculation.

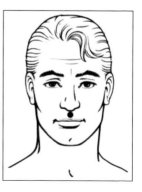

Different treatments

This section describes a series of sexual ailments with the corresponding acupressure technique for treating each one. It is advisable to apply these treatments before having sex.

Keep in mind that if the point in question is a double point, that is, it has an opposite and symmetrical point, you will need to apply pressure simultaneously to both points using both your hands. For example, if we tell you to apply pressure to double point 4 using your thumb, it means you must use the thumbs on each hand at the same time to press down on the center of each palm. Along these same lines, when a technique specifies that you must massage a double point for a certain amount of time, it is referring to the entire exercise. You must not cut the time in half.

Inhibition. Inhibitions may affect both partners and impede the free use of coitus, thereby preventing the pair from enjoying orgasm.

The causes of this problem are myriad: religious and education taboos, rejection of one's own body, psychological problems resulting in an inability to enjoy bodily pleasure, etc. To lose your inhibitions and enjoy a fulfilling and satisfying relationship in its entirety, acupressure presents several treatments.

- **First treatment.** Using the circular massage method, apply pressure to double point 17 using your thumb for two minutes. Next, rub the tips of the toes, first one and then the next, for two minutes on each foot.

- **Second treatment.** Using the middle finger of the man's right hand, touch point 1 on the woman's left foot. Do the same with the opposite hand and foot. This will transfer energy from one point to the other without the need to apply any pressure. Contact should be maintained for a prudent amount of time. Next, find individual point 8 and apply circular pressure with the index and middle fingers for two minutes. The pressure should be strong enough to drag the skin along. Then rub the tips of the toes for two minutes per foot.

■ **Third treatment.** Press down on double point 17 using the holding method for one minute. Next, apply circular pressure to individual point 8 using the index and middle fingers for two minutes hard enough to drag the skin along. Then softly rub the upper lip and the area between it and the nose for half a minute.

■ **Fourth treatment.** Press down on double point 11 using your thumb for two minutes. Then softly rub the upper lip and the area between it and the nose for half a minute.

■ **Fifth treatment.** Press down on double point 19 using the holding method for two minutes. Next, apply circular pressure to individual point 8 using the index and middle fingers for two minutes hard enough to drag the skin along.

■ **Sixth treatment.** Press down on double point 17 using the holding method for three minutes. Next, press down on double point 11 using the holding method for two minutes. To strengthen the effects of this treatment, softly rub your partner's back while applying the massage.

Lack of desire. When a couple falls into a routine, sex begins losing emotion little by little and becomes boring and not very desirable. Often, even without desire, the couple continues going through the motions and becomes trapped in a vicious circle that only creativity and a radical change in habit may break. The following treatments will help awaken the need to change those sexual habits.

■ **First treatment.** Apply pressure using the pincer method on double point 5 while adding in some easing of the pressure for two minutes. Next, with the index and middle fingers, apply circular pressure and drag the skin along on individual point 8 for a minute. Then apply pressure using the pincer method on double point 3 while adding in some easing of the pressure for a minute. Move on to rubbing the tips of the toes for a little bit, and finish by softly rubbing the base of the nape. If both partners need to recover their sexual desires, they should switch roles so that both may benefit from the massage.

■ **Second treatment.** If the man is the one lacking in sexual ardor, the woman must use her thumb to apply pressure to double point 20 and the rest of her hand to rub the sole of the foot. She will vigorously massage for two minutes. The pressure might feel slightly painful at first. Next, she will use her index and middle fingers to apply pressure to individual point 7 while using a medium amount of force for three minutes. Then she will rub the tips of the toes one by one on each foot for a couple of minutes. Finally, she will softly rub the base of the nape.

■ **Third treatment.** If the woman is the one lacking in sexual ardor, repeat the previous treatment applied to points 20 and 7, and add in two minutes of pressure to double point 39 using the thumb. Then, the man must locate points 27, 28, 29, and 30. He will passionately rub his hands down these points while at the same time nibbling his partner's lips.

Lack of energy. The stresses of modern life exhaust the body, and this tiredness affects the quality of a couple's sex life. The following treatments are very useful for toning the body before initiating coitus.

■ **First treatment.** Using your index and middle fingers, apply circular pressure to individual point 8 hard enough to drag the skin along for two minutes. Next, apply pressure in the same way to individual point 9 for half a minute. Then press down on individual point 10 in the same way as the previous two points. Finally, press down on double point 16 using the holding method for one minute.

■ **Second treatment.** Start by pressing down on double point 5 using the pincer method while adding in some easing of the pressure for about two minutes. Next, apply pressure to double point 6 using your thumb for two minutes. Finally, use the holding method to massage double point 17 for half a minute.

■ **Third treatment.** Apply pinching pressure to double point 4 for a minute by placing your thumb on the point itself and the rest of your fingers on the back of the hand. Next, use the pincer method to press down on double point 18 for one minute.

■ **Fourth treatment.** Apply pressure using the pincer method to double point 3 while adding in some easing of the pressure for two minutes. Then massage double point 20 using upward pressure toward the ankle for a minute.

■ **Fifth treatment.** Use pinching pressure to massage double point 4 by placing your thumb on the point itself and the rest of your fingers on the back of the hand for two minutes. Next, use the pincer method to massage double point 18 for one minute.

■ **Sixth treatment.** Press down on double point 16 using the holding method for two minutes. Next, massage double point 15 for two minutes, and then move on to double point 18 while applying pressure for another minute.

■ **Seventh treatment.** Press down on individual point 43 for a few seconds without moving. Afterward, turn the finger in a clockwise direction while pausing each time the recipient draws in air. Do not at any time remove the tip of your finger. Do this for a minute and a half.

■ **Eighth treatment.** This is a self-massage technique. Press down on double point 44 by joining the index finger and thumb of the same hand together and forming a small circle. This allows for the control and balance of vital energy.

Fear of the opposite sex in men. This problem generally presents itself in the later years of adolescence in young men who have had little contact with girls their age. The young man wishes to approach girls but does not because of lack of experience or shyness.

The following treatments will help conquer that fear. This massage is done in pairs.

- **First treatment.** Find double point 20 and apply pressure using the thumb. Using the rest of the hand, massage the sole of the foot, as well. The pressure must be fairly strong and might even be slightly painful to begin with. Once finished, after about five minutes, softly rub the tips of the toes on one foot and then the other for two minutes. Next, massage individual point 7. Use your index and middle fingers to apply medium pressure for about seven minutes in an uninterrupted circle while dragging the skin along. This action must reach the muscles underneath the skin.

- **Second treatment.** Find double point 20 and apply the same pressure as described in the last treatment, which is a decent amount of force. Next, press down on individual point 31 using the index and middle fingers, combining pressure and relaxation. Finish by rubbing the tips of the toes for two minutes on each foot.

- **Third treatment.** Apply pinching pressure to double point 17 for two minutes. Then find double point 5 and apply more pinching pressure and alternate it with easing of the pressure for five minutes. Finish by rubbing the tips of the toes for two minutes on each foot.

- **Fourth treatment.** Press down hard on double point 37 using your thumb for five minutes. Then find double point 5 and apply pinching pressure for two minutes.

- **Fifth treatment.** Find double point 17 and apply pinching pressure for two minutes. Next, locate double point 11 and press down with your index and middle fingers using light circular movements.

■ **Sixth treatment.** Find individual point 7 and apply a moderate amount of pressure with your index and middle fingers while dragging the skin along in an uninterrupted circle for two minutes. Next, press down firmly on double point 20 using your thumb while massaging the sole of the foot with the rest of your hand. Do this for a couple of minutes. Finish by rubbing the tips of the toes for three or four minutes.

■ **Seventh treatment.** Find double point 17 and press down using your thumb and alternate between pressure and letting up of pressure for five minutes. Next, after vigorously rubbing both feet without worrying about pressure points, continue on to double point 20 and press down using your thumb while rubbing the bottom of the foot with the rest of your hand.

Lack of control and calmness. Just as some people suffer from bulimia and eat mechanically without enjoying their food, so do some men act anxiously and recklessly during sex. This lessens their partner's enjoyment, as well as their own, and may sometimes even cause pain. For the act of sex to be enjoyable, a certain degree of calmness is required. Keep in mind that taking your time during a sexual encounter is essential. On the other hand, anxiety and the desire to move quickly will lead to premature ejaculation. If this is the case, it will be necessary to put an end to those impulses with one session (or many) of the following treatments. The woman will be acting on the man's pressure points in these massages.

■ **First treatment.** Locate double point 16, one of the gates of access to the vital energy of the orgasm, and use your thumb to apply strong pressure using circular motions and drag the skin along for three minutes. The pressure must be strong enough to affect the muscles under the skin. Next, find individual point 8 or double point 37 and apply pinching pressure for two minutes. Then use the whole palm of your hand to firmly rub the base of the nape. It is important for the man to relax and let his energy flow normally.

■ **Second treatment.** Find double point 16 and apply firm pressure using the thumb and executing a rotational motion. Drag the skin along with each movement, and allow the action to affect the muscles below the skin. Next, locate double point 17 and apply pressure for two minutes while alternating with easing of the pressure. Finally, rub the base of the nape using your entire palm for a few minutes.

■ **Third treatment.** Use your index and middle fingers to apply circular pressure to double point 22. Press down firmly and drag the skin along. Then rub the base of the nape using your entire palm for a few minutes.

■ **Fourth treatment.** Locate double point 33 and apply pressure using your left index and middle fingers in a vertical direction. Next, find double point 17 and apply pinching pressure combined with easing of the pressure for three minutes. Rub the base of the nape using your entire palm for a few minutes.

■ **Fifth treatment.** Find double point 17 and apply pinching pressure for two minutes. Then rub the base of the nape using your entire palm.

■ **Sixth Treatment.** Locate double point 16, and use your thumb to apply circular pressure for two or three minutes. Next find double point 35 and apply firm and prolonged pressure. Finally, vigorously rub the base of the nape using your entire palm.

■ **Seventh treatment.** Apply vigorous pressure to double point 37 using your thumb for two minutes. Next, locate double point 17 and press down moderately hard for two minutes while alternating between pressure and letting up of the pressure. To finish off, tenderly stroke the base of the nape using your entire palm for as long as it takes the man to relax.

■ **Eighth treatment.** Locate double point 16 under the belly button, and use your thumb to apply circular pressure for two or three minutes. Next, find double point 20 on the back of the foot and, using your thumb, apply firm pressure while massaging the bottom of the foot with the rest of your hand. To finish off, gently rub the base of the nape using your entire palm until the man is relaxed.

■ **Ninth treatment.** Vigorously apply pressure to double point 22 using your index and middle fingers for two minutes. Then find individual point 20 and apply pressure with your thumb for three minutes. Finally, rub the nape as before.

Male frigidity. Although we mostly hear about female frigidity, this problem can also affect men. Frigidity is not characterized by the lack of ejaculation but by a lack of enthusiasm during the act of sex. The man affected with frigidity participates mechanically during sex and ejaculates without any real pleasure. Frigidity must not be confused with inhibition: with the first case, the affected will glean no pleasure from masturbation or during coitus while with the second, pleasure can only be obtained through masturbation. In order to cure this unfortunate situation, we may employ these always-effective treatments.

■ **First treatment.** Use the thumb to press down on double point 17 while combining pressure and distention for two minutes. Next, find individual point 10 and apply circular pressure with the index and middle fingers for two minutes. The pressure should be strong enough to drag the skin along. Finally, softly rub the tips of the toes one by one for two minutes.

■ **Second treatment.** Find double point 20 and apply pressure with your thumb for one minute. Then rub the tips of the toes one by one for two minutes.

■ **Third treatment.** Firmly press down on double point 20 with your thumb for one minute. Next, locate individual point 7, one of the gates of access to the vital energies of the human body, and press down using your index and middle fingers. The pressure should be strong enough to drag the skin along in a circular motion so that the action may affect the muscles under the skin. Finally, rub the tips of the toes, first one and then the next, for two minutes.

■ **Fourth treatment.** Locate double point 21 and press down with your thumb using the pincer method for one minute. Next, find double point 20 and apply firm pressure with the thumb for one minute. Finally, rub the tips of the toes one by one for two minutes.

■ **Fifth treatment.** Locate double point 21 and press down with your thumb using the pincer method for one minute. Find individual point 7 and press down using your index and middle fingers hard enough to drag the skin along in a circular motion for the muscles underneath to be affected. Finally, rub the tips of the toes, first one and then the next, for two minutes.

■ **Sixth treatment.** Find double point 20 and apply firm and decisive pressure with your thumb for one minute. Afterward, locate double point 6 and apply pressure with your thumb for two minutes. To finish off, press down on point 20 again for another two minutes.

■ **Seventh treatment.** Find double point 17 and press down using your thumb while alternating between pressure and letting up of the pressure for three minutes. Next, find individual point 8 and apply circular pressure with the index and middle fingers for two minutes. The pressure should be strong enough to drag the skin along. Finally, use your thumbs to massage point 1 for two minutes.

■ **Eighth treatment.** Repeat the previous treatment and accompany the final massage with sensual strokes over the whole body, paying special attention to the legs. Before initiating sex, massage double point 3 for five minutes using your thumbs.

Premature ejaculation. In this section, we will outline a number of treatments for curing premature ejaculation. The treatments may also be applied in cases of early ejaculation, which differs from premature ejaculation in that it happens before penetration.

The length of the sexual act varies greatly from man to man, which makes it difficult to establish an average that may be used to identify premature ejaculation. And so we will say that an act of sex that does not last long enough happens when the male ejaculates before the female orgasms. This problem occurs when the man tends to reach sexual ecstasy sooner than the woman and shortly after penetration. It is important to note that the diagnosis may only be given in a situation where the problem repeats itself. If there are only isolated cases, there is no reason to call it a case of premature ejaculation.

Taoism has come up with many methods for beating premature ejaculation because it proposes that the woman's pleasure is very beneficial for the man's health. Additionally, it is thought that the man must be able to control his ejaculation and separate it from orgasm in order to fortify his being. In ancient China, any man who suffered from this problem was considered sexually immature. If you fall into this category, do not hesitate to use the following treatments.

■ **First treatment.** Find double point 17 and press down using your thumb. Apply light circular pressure for two minutes. Next, find double point 10 and press down using your middle finger. Alternate between pressure and easing of the pressure for five minutes. Once finished and after a brief rest, you may verify the efficacy of the treatment by having sex. If during penetration the man feels that he is about to ejaculate before the woman has had a chance, he should withdraw his penis from the vagina, breathe abdominally, and reapply pressure to point 10.

■ **Second treatment.** Find double point 17 and apply pressure using the holding method while alternating between pressure and the easing of pressure for five minutes.

■ **Third treatment.** Find double point 17 and apply pinching pressure for two minutes. Next, find double point 23 and apply pressure using your index and middle fingers without rotating them for a minute. Next, press down on double point 24 in the same manner as you have just done to point 23.

■ **Fourth treatment.** Locate individual point 9 and apply pressure using your index and middle fingers. Alternate between pressure and the easing of pressure using moderate force for two minutes. Next, find double point 23 and press down while combining pressure and the easing of pressure for two minutes. Lastly, apply pressure to individual point 8 in the same way as you have just done to point 9 for the same amount of time.

■ **Fifth treatment.** Locate individual point 8 and apply pressure using your index and middle fingers. Alternate between pressure and the easing of pressure while using moderate force for two minutes. Next, find double point 17 and press down while combining pressure and the easing of pressure for two minutes.

■ **Sixth treatment.** Premature ejaculation may also be cured with frequent and energetic massages combining pressure and the easing of pressure on the epigastric region (the area of the abdomen located between the sternum, belly button, and false ribs) and the sacrum. This same exercise may help more mature men to perform coitus several times with only one ejaculation to ensure that the loss of semen is minimized and there is no exhaustion.

■ **Seventh treatment.** Reapply the first treatment, and add in a massage to double point 3 using your thumb. Combine pressure and the easing of pressure for several minutes. Repeat this last massage as many times as needed.

■ **Eighth treatment.** This treatment, unlike the rest, which should be done before initiating sex, is to be applied during coitus and is used to keep from ejaculating before the woman has reached orgasm. When the man feels that he is going to ejaculate, he should pull his penis out of the vagina and he or the woman must hold the gland with one hand and firmly press down on the frenulum using the thumb. This technique should be applied as many times as needed.

■ **Ninth treatment.** Locate individual point 43 and apply constant pressure in the direction of the lower part of the nose. Maintain this pressure for four minutes. This treatment bolsters the body's regulation of *Yin* and *Yang*. It is the imbalance of these energies that causes premature ejaculation.

Impotence. Impotence may have psychological or physical causes or a mix of both. Among the psychological reasons for impotence, we have stress, tiredness, loss of self esteem, fear of failure, anxiety, traumatic experiences, etc. Physical causes for this condition may include injuries to the central nervous system (paralysis, inflammations, trauma, etc.), intoxication (alcohol, heroin, cocaine, etc.), diabetes, endocrine disruptions or lesions, etc.

Impotence may present itself in a number of ways to greater and lesser extents: complete absence of erection, unstable erections (do not last long enough to finish coitus), insufficient erections (the penis does not become stiff enough to penetrate the vagina), and unpredictable erections (they disappear at random without any seeming cause that may explain why). A person may only be diagnosed as suffering from impotence if their erectile problems are consistent and always present.

The following treatments are of great use against psychological impotence. In order for the treatment to be effective, one needs the cooperation of their female sexual companion, as well as a positive and carefree attitude. The patient should relax and let their body react as it will.

These treatments, unlike others, should be done independently of sex. You should not take advantage of any erections produced during the treatment to have sex. You will need to first successfully complete the treatment over several days before being able to have sex after the massage.

- **First treatment.** Locate individual point 8 and apply circular pressure using the index and middle fingers for half a minute. Point 8 is the most important pressure point in treating impotence for acupuncture, as well as acupressure. Next, find double point 18 and press down using the pincer method for another half of a minute. Finally, locate double point 16 and apply pressure by holding tightly.

- **Second treatment.** Locate individual point 8 and apply circular pressure using the index and middle fingers for a minute. Then locate double point 17 and apply pressure by holding tightly for two minutes.

- **Third treatment.** Press down on individual point 8 using your index and middle fingers with enough strength to drag the skin along with each rotation for a minute. Next find double point 17 and apply holding pressure for two minutes. Then locate double point 16 and apply pressure in the same manner as the last point. Finally, locate double point 23 and apply pressure with your thumb for about one minute.

- **Fourth treatment.** Locate individual point 8 and apply circular pressure using the index and middle fingers for a minute. Then locate double point 17 and apply pressure by holding tightly for about three minutes. Finally, find double point 16 and apply pressure for one minute.

■ **Fifth treatment.** Locate double point 20 and apply pressure with your thumb for two minutes. Next find double point 12 and apply circular pressure using the index and middle fingers for one minute. Finally, find double point 16 and apply holding pressure for one minute.

■ **Sixth treatment.** Locate double point 23 and apply pressure with your thumb for one minute. Locate individual point 8 and apply circular pressure using the index and middle fingers for three minutes. Finish by applying pressure to double point 3 for a couple of minutes.

Fear of the male gender. As with men, women may also have problems communicating sexually with the opposite sex. This is common in adolescent girls who may have had little contact with boys their age. The problem may be exacerbated by an excessively rigid education that excessively underscores the differences between the sexes while imposing norms and taboos. This may make it difficult to engage in sexual activity. To solve the problem, it is necessary to increase trust between the couple.

These treatments help banish the woman's fears and, in order to be effective, require the complete collaboration of the man, who must be gentle with his sexual partner and soothe her with sweet words. This will allow her to feel relaxed and enjoy herself during coitus.

■ **First treatment.** Locate double point 17 on the female body and apply pressure using the thumbs while massaging the back of the legs with the rest of your hands for two minutes. Next, softly rub the tips of the toes, first one and then the next, for three minutes on each foot.

■ **Second treatment.** Find double point 18 and apply pressure using the pinching method while spending three minutes on each ankle. Then rub the tips of the toes for three minutes on each foot.

■ **Third treatment.** Locate double point 17 and apply pressure by pinching for three minutes on each ankle. Next, find double point 11 and apply pressure using your index and middle fingers while rotating lightly for five minutes. Finish by rubbing the tips of the toes.

■ **Fourth treatment.** Locate double point 5 and apply pressure with your thumb for five minutes. At the end of this lapse of time, use your thumbs to massage double point 3 for two minutes.

■ **Fifth treatment.** Locate double point 18 and massage it using the pinching method for two minutes. Next, softly rub the tips of the toes, first one and then the next, for another two minutes. Finally, find double point 5 and apply firm pressure with your thumbs for one minute.

■ **Sixth treatment.** Find double point 20 and press down using your thumb for three minutes. Use the rest of your hand to massage the bottom of the foot. Next, find double point 17 and apply pressure using your thumbs while massaging the back of the leg with the rest of your hand for three minutes.

■ **Seventh treatment.** Locate double point 17 and use the same style of pressure and amount of time as the last treatment. Finally, find double point 5 and apply pressure with your thumb for three minutes.

■ **Eighth treatment.** The man's right middle finger must come into contact with point 1 on the woman's left foot. Then the man must do the same with his opposite finger and the woman's opposite foot. By holding this position, both of their energies will become balanced. Finish this treatment by repeating the previous treatment.

Female frigidity. There are two kinds of frigidity. The first happens when there is a complete absence of sexual arousal following correct stimulation. That is to say, there is no lubrication, quickening of the pulse, etc. This may be considered the female equivalent of male impotence, and as with the man, the causes could be physical or psychological. With the second kind of frigidity, there may be physical signs of sexual arousal, but the woman does not feel pleasure during the act of sex.

Be careful not to confuse female frigidity with male premature ejaculation. If the man initiates sex too soon without paying attention to the signs, reactions, and wishes of the woman, she will not be ready for coitus and will not enjoy it.

Keep in mind that any woman who feels pleasure through masturbating is not considered to be suffering from frigidity. If a woman experiences pleasure by herself but not during a correctly realized sexual session with her partner, we are faced with a problem of inhibition not frigidity.

If we are dealing with a mistaken case of frigidity, the cause usually lies with the man, who is not correctly stimulating his partner. In this case, the following exercises will be ineffective. If we are dealing with a real case of frigidity, it may be cured by using the following treatments.

■ **First treatment.** Find double point 17 and apply pinching pressure for a couple of minutes.

■ **Second treatment.** Locate double point 21 and press down with the tip of your right thumb using the pinching method. Next, find individual point 8 and apply circular pressure with the index and middle fingers. The pressure should be strong enough to drag the skin along.

■ **Third treatment.** Locate double point 19 and apply pressure using the pincer method for two minutes. Next, find double point 17 and apply holding pressure for two minutes. Finally, locate double point 2 and apply gentle pressure at a 45 degree angle with the bridge of the nose.

■ **Fourth treatment.** Find individual point 12 and apply circular pressure with the index and middle fingers. The pressure should be strong enough to drag the skin along. Next, find double point 16 and apply holding pressure for three minutes. Then find double point 13 and press down using your index and middle fingers hard enough to drag the skin along in a circular motion and for the muscles underneath to be affected. Next, press down on double point 15 exactly in the same way as with point 16 and for the same amount of time. Finally, apply pressure to double point 17 using the same method and amount of time as with point 16.

■ **Fifth treatment.** Find double point 39 and apply strong pressure for two minutes. Gently move your hands upward along points 27, 28, 29, and 30. Finally, locate double point 17 and apply pressure for two minutes while stroking the ankle.

■ **Sixth treatment.** Locate double point 17 and apply pressure using the holding method for two minutes. Finish by firmly massaging double point 19 with your thumbs for another three minutes.

■ **Seventh treatment.** Locate points 27, 28, 29, and 30, and rub your hands gently up and down them while increasing pressure with each pass. Then firmly press down on point 1. Next, find double point 15 and apply holding pressure. Kind and tender words will aid in the effectiveness of this treatment.

■ **Eighth treatment.** Locate double point 19 and apply pressure using the pincer method for three minutes. Next, find double point 16 and apply holding pressure for another three minutes.

■ **Ninth treatment.** Repeat the previous treatment and accompany it with sensual caresses across the whole body, thereby prolonging the process until the woman expresses a desire to initiate sex.

■ **Tenth treatment.** Press down on individual point 43 for a few seconds without moving. Afterward, turn the finger in a clockwise direction while pausing each time the woman draws in air. Do not at any time remove the tip of your finger. Do this for a minute and a half.

Fear of experiencing pain during penetration. The fear of experiencing pain during penetration may by motivated by a lack of knowledge (for example, if this is the first time having sex) or by past unenjoyable experiences (for example, if pain was experienced after initiating coitus before the woman was well lubricated or if the man was not in control of himself), among other things.

This fear may come to prevent penetration or the receiving of pleasure during sex. To avoid it, it is necessary to do the following treatments before initiating coitus. It is also advisable that the woman be on top of the man during the sexual act so that she may be the one in control of the depth and angle of penetration.

The man should seek to soothe these fears using gentle caresses and tender words that inspire trust.

■ **First treatment.** Find individual point 9 and apply circular pressure with the index and middle fingers for a minute and a half. The pressure should be strong enough to drag the skin along. Next, find double point 18 and press down using the pincer method for another minute.

■ **Second treatment.** Locate double point 18 and apply pressure using the pincer method. Next, press down on individual point 9 using your index and middle fingers with enough strength to drag the skin along with each rotation for a minute. Finally, locate individual point 8 and apply pressure similarly to how you did it in the last part.

■ **Third treatment.** Locate double point 18 and apply pressure using the pincer method. Finish by locating double point 30 and applying pressure with your thumb for two minutes.

- **Fourth treatment.** Find double point 18 and apply pinching pressure for two minutes. Next, locate individual point 9 and apply circular pressure using the index and middle fingers for two minutes.

- **Fifth treatment.** Locate double point 18 and apply pressure using the pincer method for two minutes. Next, find individual point 23 and apply circular pressure combined with the letting up of pressure for one minute.

- **Sixth treatment.** The man's right middle finger must come into contact with point 1 on the woman's left foot. Then the man must do the same with his opposite finger and the woman's opposite foot. Hold this position without exerting any pressure. Before penetration, the man must show himself to be loving and will massage the woman's feet by holding them in his hands and applying gentle pressure in order to fill her with trust.

Feminine and masculine energy

Alongside the energy of the Universe, Taoists also believe in physical or environmental energies, such as breathing, feeding, and solar energy, as well as other more subtle ones. We inherit our sexual energy from our parents at the time of conception (*Ching Chi,* or primordial vital energy) and it is one of the basic forces that maintains us throughout our lives. Once it dries up, we die.

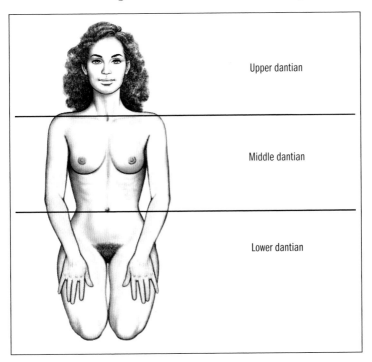

Upper dantian

Middle dantian

Lower dantian

Taoists acknowledge the existence of three cores of divine energy. The lower core is situated in the pelvic and abdominal region. That is where we store and replenish our energy, power, and sexual vitality. The middle core, in the pectoral area, is where we conserve and rekindle our passion, courage, and emotions. Finally, in the upper core, the head and brain, we gather and renew the manifestation of our conscious and spiritual energy, as well as our intellect.

If the energy that flows through our bodies becomes blocked, we tend to breathe shallowly, which restricts the flow of blood and other fluids, creating tension (in our back and abdomen) and stiffening our diaphragm, which acts as a valve between the upper and lower dantians. In order to open this valve, it is necessary to breathe deeply and calmly, which, along with different massages, allows us to open the paths for our sexual energy. As it flows, this energy sets flame to our passions and the desire to brighten our thoughts and renew the three fields of energy.

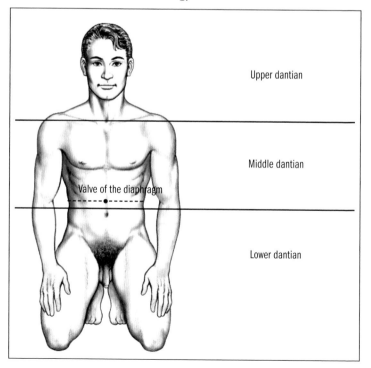

Upper dantian

Middle dantian

Valve of the diaphragm

Lower dantian

Taoists believe that our very existence is the product of the interaction between *Yin* energy (female) and *Yang* energy (male). And so they realized thousands of years before modern Western scientific society that the polarity between the sexes exists at every level, down to the cells, and that a delicate balance of hormones, male or female, determines the sexual identity of each person.

Also, the sexual coexistence between each couple allows one to understand, according to *Tao*, that the man or woman with whom each person lives corresponds, or is very similar to, the spiritual opposite: manifestations of divine essence in search of unity.

Chinese aphrodisiac food

The Tao that can be known is not the Tao.
The substance of the world is only one name for the Tao.
The Tao is everything that exists and could exist.
The world is but a map of what exists and could exist...

During antiquity, men observed the plants. They watched an orange grow and, seven moons later, saw how its seeds become succulent fruits themselves. From these observations were born the beliefs that would guide the first brewers of aphrodisiac potions. They thought that if the root of a plant resembled genitalia, they would have a stimulating effect and inside them could be found a wonderful fruit, the source of eternal pleasure.

And so the search began. Chinese wise men searched for substances that would light the flame of passion and increase sexual appetite. They went into the mountains and dedicated themselves to look for plants that might hold these splendid secrets. And so during about the fifth millennium B.C., they discovered a root that, aside from possessing curative properties and bolstering longevity, could be used as a sexual stimulant: ginseng. This discovery spread to India, where the sacred texts of Hinduism now speak of its beneficial qualities. They also found ginger, the pulpy fruit and aromatic stem of which they thought might incite a great pleasure in men. They were also captivated by a brown-colored fruit with a hard outer layer that contained inside it two fleshy halves separated by a membrane. And so they began using nutmeg.

By collecting roots and seeds, the Chinese discovered little by little the powerful aphrodisiacs that were gifted to them by nature herself, benevolent in her wish to give up her secrets. Women, like patient artisans, began learning the secrets of the plants and made of them an atavistic legacy that they eventually applied to Chinese cooking.

There are still Chinese recipes today that increase sexual potency and ignite erotic desire. Below you will find the ingredients and methods for preparing these foods. They will undoubtedly satisfy you.

Frog legs

Ingredients
2 dozen frog legs
2 Tbsp of ginger, finely chopped
2 Tbsp of rice wine
2 Tbsp of water
2 chili peppers, finely chopped
6 green peppers, chopped
2 garlic cloves
¼ cup of oil for frying
1 Tbsp of soy beans
A few drops of sesame oil

Preparation
Heat the oil in a sauté pan over medium heat, and fry the frog legs for about two minutes.

Remove part of the oil, leaving about three tablespoons, and sauté the chili peppers, garlic, ginger, and soy beans. Toss in the green peppers. Finally, add the water mixture, the sesame oil, and the wine. Bring to a boil for a few seconds and then remove the pan from the heat. Serve immediately with rice or a salad.

Abalones on a bed of lettuce

Ingredients
2 Tbsp of oil
About 1lb (½ kg) of mushrooms
About 1lb (½ kg) of abalones, sliced

The sauce
6 chunks of ginger, cut into strips
6 scallions
1 head of lettuce
1 Tbsp of soy sauce
2 Tbsp of sesame oil
1 Tbsp of sugar
1 Tbsp of cornstarch

Preparation
Cut the mushrooms in half, and boil the lettuce in water for one minute. Remove the lettuce, drain well, and place in the bottom of a dish.

Heat the oil in a pan and, once it is hot, toss in the onion chives, mushrooms, and ginger.

Once the vegetables have been sautéed, add the abalones, sauté some more, and then add the rest of the sauce ingredients. Once the sauce has thickened, pour the entire mixture onto the bed of lettuce.

Note: If abalones are not available, you may substitute them with scallops.

Ginger rabbit

Ingredients
About 1lb (½ kg) of rabbit, diced
2 Tbsp of ginger, finely chopped

Olive oil
12-oz (33 cl) bottle of beer
Salt
Pepper

Preparation

Wash and drain the rabbit well. Heat the oil in a pan and fry the ginger. Let the oil cool down a bit, and then add the rabbit and beer. Simmer on low heat until there is no liquid left. Season with salt and pepper to taste.

Spring rolls

Ingredients

5 Tbsp of flour
1 egg, beaten, plus 1 additional egg to seal the spring rolls
1 teaspoon of salt
8 oz (225 g) of veal, chopped
3 onions, chopped
7 oz (220 g) of cabbage, chopped
3½ oz (100 g) of prawns, shredded
Oil

Preparation

To make the dough for the rolls, mix the flour, egg, and salt together. Knead the mixture, and let it sit in the fridge overnight. The next morning, knead the dough again, and then roll it out with a rolling pin until it is very thin. Heat a saute pan over medium heat with 2 tablespoons of oil and fry the meat for 4 to 6 minutes. Add in the onion, cabbage, and prawns. Season and sauté for ten minutes. Drain the mixture and let it cool. Cut the dough in squares, and fill each square with the prawn mixture. Roll the dough up and seal the edges up with the egg. Deep fry the rolls in oil until they turn golden and crispy.

Shanghai chicken

Ingredients
8 chicken thighs
2 Tbsp of soy sauce
2 Tbsp of cooking sherry
1 pinch of sugar
About 5 oz. (150 g) of peas
17½ oz. (500 g) of mushrooms, cut in half
1 onion
2 cups of tomatoes, crushed
2 Tbsp of oil
Salt
Ginger
Pepper

Preparation
In a bowl, mix together the chicken thighs, soy sauce, sherry, salt, sugar, pepper, and ginger. Let the chicken marinade.

Heat the oil in a pan and fry the mushrooms and the onions. Season with salt. Drain the mushrooms and onions and add the chicken mixture to the leftover oil. Cover the pan and simmer on low heat for ten minutes. Add the mushrooms and onions, tomatoes, and peas. Stir and serve when hot.

Fried rice with shrimp

Ingredients
2 Tbsp of oil
2 onions
About 1lb (½ kg) of shrimp
About 1lb (½ kg) of mushrooms
3 Tbsp of soy sauce
2 cups of cooked rice
1 egg, beaten

Salt
Pepper

Preparation

Heat the oil in a pan and sauté the onions and shrimp for three minutes. Add the pepper, salt, mushrooms, soy sauce, and rice. Pour in the egg and stir over low heat for 2 to 4 minutes.

Braised prawns

Ingredients

8 oz. (225 g) of raw prawns
2 tsp of sherry or rice wine
1 tsp of salt
1 tsp of green onion, finely chopped
2 tsp of ginger
½ tsp of cornstarch mixed with ½ tsp of water

Preparation

Peel and devein the prawns. Wash them and let them dry on a paper towel. Pour all the other ingredients into a large pan. Bring the mixture to a boil, and then add the prawns. Braise them over low heat for 3 or 4 minutes. Serve immediately.

Sichuan crispy duck

Ingredients

1 whole duck
2 Tbsp of five spice powder
2 Tbsp of salt
4 chunks of fresh ginger
4 green onions
34 oz. (1 l) of peanut oil
1 cup of water

Preparation

Thaw the duck if it is frozen and leave it to dry. Once dry, rub the inside and outside of the duck with salt and five spice powder. Wrap the duck in plastic wrap, and let it sit in the fridge for at least three hours. After the duck has had time to sit, cut the ginger and the green onions into large chunks. Fill the inside of the duck with the ginger and green onions, and place it in a heat-resistant dish. In a pot, large enough to fit the duck entirely, place a circular wire rack. Place the duck on the rack and only add enough water to reach the bottom of the duck. Bring the water to a boil and place the lid on the pot. Be sure to add more water, as it will evaporate as the duck cooks. Steam the duck for two hours. Take the duck out and throw out any extra fat along with the pieces of ginger and green onion. Store the duck in the refrigerator for a couple of hours until it is cool and dry.

Before serving, slice the duck. Heat the peanut oil in a pot, and fry the slices until they are crispy.

Roasted quail

Ingredients
6 whole quails, about 3½ oz. (100 g) each
1 tablespoon of salt

The sauce
1 Tbsp of rice wine or sherry
1 Tbsp of clear soy sauce

Preparation
Preheat the oven to 464° F (240° C). If the quail are frozen, be sure to completely thaw them beforehand. Once they are totally dry, rub them inside and out with salt. Place the birds in the oven for 5 minutes. After 5 minutes, lower the temperature to 356° F (180° C) and continue roasting for 20 minutes. Turn the oven off and leave the quails in for another 5 minutes. Take the quail out and let them rest for 10 minutes. Add the sauce and serve.

Epilogue

The hands are a powerful tool. They may be used to stroke, convey love, communicate, and heal. A caress of the hand can be used as therapy, and human contact becomes physical and spiritual healing. They help us speak without words and, through them, we can achieve spiritual understanding by making energy flow through the inside of our organism.

Using this book, you can become an authentic acupressurist by practicing the art of healing with your hands. Pleasing your partner will not only benefit them. You, too, will be able to open the doors to a world full of sensations and positive energy, become closer to your partner, gain their trust, and create a state of well-being that is both physical and emotional. All these things are possible once you learn and practice these thousand-year-old techniques.

The techniques of therapeutic massage using acupuncture points and the energy meridians have been used in China for the past two thousand years. This millennial practice is based on traditional theories that massaging and applying pressure to certain points on the body eases the flow of energy through the interior and heals internal organs of disease.

Acupressure is the medicinal technique that may be applied to diverse ailments. It is the same as acupuncture except it makes use of the hands. This should bring joy to those people who, for some reason or other, fear needles and believe that they will be hurt by them. Acupressure also offers us the chance to become our own master, that is to say to learn the art of healing massage by ourselves without needing to turn to a center of learning.

This is the purpose of this book: to provide you with all the information necessary to delve into the secrets of erotic massage and acupressure. You may feel clumsy at first and take a little more time than you would want to locate the specific points on the body. You must not worry; patience and the will to learn will be your allies, and the great benefits you will enjoy will be motivation enough for you to become an expert in massage.

Remember that sexuality is more than just a physical act. When you rid yourself of your clothes to become closer to your partner, you rid yourself, also, of your problems and the tension in your body, and you let your love become an exchange of physical and spiritual energy.

Bibliography

ANAND, Margo. *La senda del éxtasis*. Ed. Martínez Roca. Barcelona, 1990

CHANG, Jolan. *El Tao del amor y del sexo*. Ed. Plaza&Janés. Barcelona, 1971

CHIA, Mantak; CHIA, Maneewan; ABRAMS, Douglas and CARL-TON, Rachel. *La pareja multiorgásmica*. Neo Person Editions. Madrid, 2000

CHIA, Mantak y ARAVA, Douglas. *El hombre multiorgásmico*. Neo Person Editions. Madrid, 1999

CHUANGUI, Wang. *Digitopuntura china*. Oceano-Ibis. Barcelona, 1995

FERRARA, Guillermo. *Manual de masaje holístico*. Océano Ambar. Barcelona, 2002

HENG, Cheng. *El Tao del amor*. Apóstrofe Editions. Barcelona, 1999

HSI LAI. *Enseñanzas sexuales de la tigresa blanca*. Obelisco Editions. Barcelona, 2003

RUSSELL, Stephen y Kolb, Jürgen. *El Tao del masaje sexual*. Integral. Barcelona, 1992

TSE, Lao. *Tao Te Ching. El libro clásico de la sabiduría china*. Integral. Barcelona, 1995

TSAI SU-UN, Hsuan. *Puntos del placer. La digitopuntura sexual*. Ed. Martínez Roca. Barcelona, 2002

ORTEGA, Natalia. *Amar toda la noche*. Océano Ambar. Barcelona, 2000

VAN GULIK, R.H. *La vida sexual en la antigua china*. Ed. Siruela. Madrid, 2000

YU-TANG, Wu. *Guía del masaje erótico*. Obelisco Editions. Barcelona, 1999